Not Somehow

David Banks was born in Hull. He is an actor with many TV and theatre roles to his credit. In BBC's *Doctor Who* he portrayed the Cyberleader throughout the 1980's, and played the obsessive lawyer Graeme Curtis in *Brookside*. His first published book was *Cybermen* – which has been described as an insider's guide to the Cyber race. With Janice Cramer he compiled another sort of guide – for actors in search of accommodation: the *Good Digs Guide*. His play *Severance* was performed as part of the London New Play Festival. *Duke in Darkness* is his adaptation of Patrick Hamilton's wartime play of the same title. *Iceberg*, David's first novel, was published in 1993 by Virgin. He lives in Islington.

Mina Banks SRN SCM RNT received general, midwifery and district nursing training at St Mary's Hospital, Islington. She was staff nurse and ward sister at a London children's hospital, trained in tropical diseases and hospital housekeeping and was sister in charge of Eye, Gynaecological and Theatre departments at the Kent and Sussex Hospital, Tunbridge Wells. In the early years of the Second World War she was appointed matron at the King George V Hospital in Malta during the siege of the island. Returning to England she ran the Barnardo's John Capel Hanbury Hospital for six years and during her matronship established an affiliated School of Nursing with two London teaching hospitals. Following work at the National Hospital for Nervous Diseases and at Beckenham Hospital, Kent, Mina took a sister tutor diploma at Hull University and stayed in the city to teach nursing, first as sister tutor, then as principal tutor at the Western General Hospital. In 1964 she became Deputy Principal of the Hull School of Nursing, a post she held until her retirement. She has been examiner to the United Sheffield Hospitals, examiner to the General Nursing Council since 1944, member of its Moderating Committee and of the Hull Health Council Committee and key member of the Royal College of Nursing. She was President of the Hull Soroptimists and the St John's Ambulance Brigade (Hull Combined Eastern Division), founder member and President of the Western General Hospital League, and General Secretary of the Hull Ladies Musical Union. She now lives in the village of Swanland, North Humberside.

Not Somehow

the story of a Christian life in nursing

Mina Banks

told in her own words
with the help of
David Banks

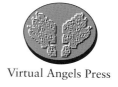

Virtual Angels Press

NOT SOMEHOW

First published in the United Kingdom in 1995 by
Virtual Angels Press
67c St Peter's Street London N1 8JR

Not Somehow is a work of reconstructed memory and
should not be read as a document of historical fact

The photographs on pages 107, 115, 129, 133 and 145
are courtesy of Hull Daily Mail Publications Ltd

British Library Cataloguing in Publication Data
A catalogue record for this book is available
from the British Library

ISBN 0 9526303 0 3

Printed in the United Kingdom by Biddles Limited
Woodbridge Park, Guildford, Surrey GU1 1DA

For Douglas

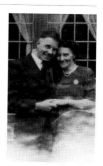

Contents

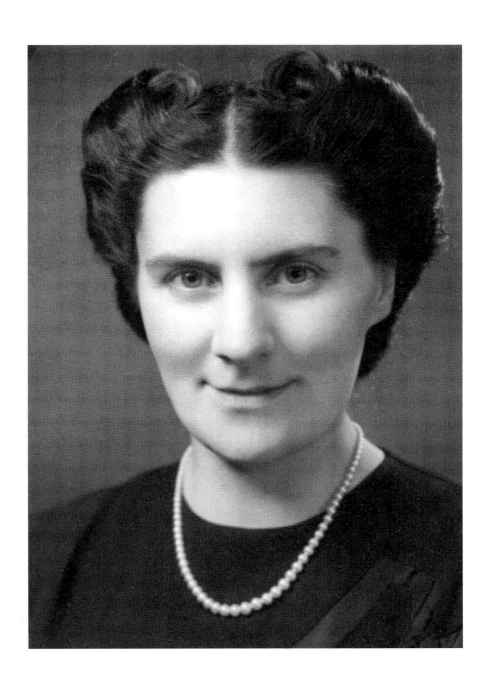

Foreword

Mina Banks has had a remarkable life. Born Mina Staerck into a large family in 1908 and orphaned at four years old, she became a Christian in her teens and trained as a nurse so that she could be a missionary in China. But she failed the medical and instead embarked on a life of nursing service that took her to a London mission, a Barnardo's Home, to Malta during the war, and then to Hull, where she met and married Douglas Banks, taught as a sister tutor, and eventually became Deputy Principal of the Hull School of Nursing.

I first met her, and Douglas, in 1975 when I joined the church they attended in Hull. I soon came to know them as a friendly and hospitable couple with a warm Christian faith. I knew little more about them until one day in 1980 I received a message to say that Mina had suffered a major stroke and was in a deep coma. I went at once to the hospital where I learnt that the doctor had given Douglas and their son David little hope that she would recover. Seeing her, I could only feel that the doctor was right. Yet remarkably she regained consciousness and, together with Douglas and David, began a long fight to cope with the paralysis her stroke had caused.

In this fight Mina and Douglas drew upon all the resources of their Christian faith. It became a source of inspiration to me to see them casting themselves upon the Lord and drawing strength from Him. I began to learn how they had come to have such faith – from the days of their conversion, through the experiences of their early Christian lives, until they met each other in 1949 and fell in love.

In 1993 Mina lost Douglas. He was very nearly ninety-one and had striven to the last in determined and devoted care for Mina. Since then she has had to dig deeper still into her spiritual resources. I continue to be impressed by the way she keeps going, keeps cheerful, keeps thinking of others, keeps trusting her Saviour. Her memoirs are a moving testimony to this.

Mina's is a story of struggle and faith, spanning almost the whole of the century. It provides an insight into the extraordinary lives of ordinary people. But more than this, her story gives heart to those of us who are struggling with difficulties and disappointments in our own lives as we try to believe that to those who love God all things *do* work together for good.

Dr Peter Nelson
University of Hull
May 1995

Co-Author's Note and Acknowledgements

Over the past eight years I have been helping my mother write the story of her life. This book is the result. But in truth her story has been eighty-seven years in the making – the years of my mother's life.

The effects of a stroke made it difficult for her to write her story down, though she did at first attempt it. She found it easier to record her recollections on tape. She has a gift for recounting events verbatim and an impressive memory for detail. Her storytelling has a direct, simple style which I have tried to preserve. The narrative has been shaped from these recollections to form the eighteen chapters of the book.

Each chapter is preceded by a short quotation from the Bible. These are taken from the Revised Standard Version. Passages of the Bible within the text are from the King James Version. The book referred to in the final chapter, *Before and After Cannizzaro* by Dr John Bradley, is published by Whittles (Latheronwheel, 1992).

The *Hull Daily Mail* has from time to time covered the professional activities with which my mother has been involved. I would like to thank the present editor and director Michael G Wood for his kind permission to reproduce some of the pictures of my mother taken by his newspaper over the last forty years.

In 1973 Barbara Robinson (also known as columnist Jane Humber of the Hull Daily Mail) published an interview to mark my mother's retirement. It was Barbara's positive response at that time which planted the seed in my mother's mind that her life story might sometime make the basis of a book. My mother wishes now to acknowledge that inspiration.

Grateful acknowledgement is also due to Pat Glaholm and Kathryn Bird, my mother's carers, who have supported her with patient affection and dedicated concern; quite simply, they have made it possible for my mother to remain at home and so complete her story.

The faithfulness of her close friends Peter Nelson, Grace and Kenneth Gibbs, and Rupert Griffin can never be adequately expressed. Without their Christian fellowship her recent years would have been much the poorer.

Likewise, there are a host of others – too many to include them all here – who have kept her spirits high through their regular visits, encouragement and practical support. Individual mention must be made of John Glaholm and his care of the garden, Patricia Griffiths and her life-enhancing aromatherapy skills, Dave Green and his invaluable taxi service, Samantha and Lyndsey and their father Richard Bird, Mary Gorman, Joan Cooper, Meg and Brian Deakin and their little dog Benjy, Marianne Tansey and her son – my mother's godson – Christopher Tansey, Thelma Carter and the Quarry Bank Nursing Home, Maureen Wilson and Sally Bell and the Humberside Social Services, Mrs Lamb and the Swanland Library, and Sister Mary Moody, Linda Trotter, Jill Craik and the other district nurses whose care and involvement have far exceeded the demands of professional duty.

John Wells – my mother's other godson – very kindly found time to read the manuscript and correct some errors of historical fact. Peter Nelson also read the manuscript, making helpful corrections, and Maureen Purkis spent many hours of diligent proofreading at all stages of the book's development. My heartfelt thanks to each of them.

Above all, acknowledgement must go to my father, who for more than forty years was the mainstay of my mother's life, and who for the last, hard, thirteen years of his life gave to her devotion and support beyond what seemed humanly possible and, finally, beyond what it was his to give.

A card accompanying some flowers for my parents' wedding day bore the words: 'Not somehow but triumphantly'. The card was stuck in the frame of a wedding photo, and as I grew up the initial strangeness of this phrase became familiar to me. In the course of writing this book, as the pattern of her story emerged more clearly, those words seemed also to describe her life and Christian belief. The constant underlying theme of her memoirs is God's faithfulness; how He led her in ways that were beyond her understanding at the time, but that later made a clearer sense. Things did not happen any old how. The unfolding of events was planned. The difficulties and disappointments, as well as the times of success and happiness, were part of a greater purpose.

Not somehow but triumphantly. This is her deep conviction. Hence the title of this book – *Not Somehow* – my mother's eighty-seven year long story.

David Banks
Islington
July 1995

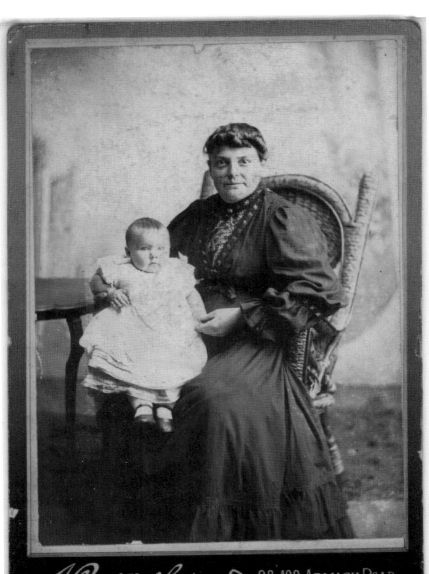

A. Griffiths & Sons. STUDIO   98-100 ARMAGH ROAD
NORTH BOW.

1

My Early Life

Like newborn babes, long for the pure spiritual milk,
that by it you may grow up to salvation;
for you have tasted the kindness of the Lord.
1 Peter 2.2-3

I was born prematurely on the eleventh of March 1908.

My weight was two pounds exactly. Since I was so tiny and fragile my mother clothed me in soft fabric and had me lying on a silk-covered pillow with instructions to the family that only she might touch me.

I was baptised in a soup bowl.

The name I was christened with was Minnie. But my brother Edward, six years old, would creep up to my cradle when he thought no one was watching, and would stroke my tiny arms and face, and would croon over me, 'Minnie, minnie, mina!'. That was how I came to be known as Mina.

At six months old I developed pneumonia and was carried to the Great London Hospital by my mother. I have a recollection of being carried up and round many stairs, crying. When I mentioned this to my eldest sister, Alice, many years later, and described to her the white tiles, she was amazed. 'You were so small,' she said. 'Yes, you were taken by our mother and cried all the way up the stairs.' Much later on, in the course of my work as a nurse, I visited the hospital and saw for myself those stairs and the white tiles.

I was the youngest of seven. Eddie was my youngest brother and Alice was my oldest sister. Then there were my much older brothers, William and Arthur, and my other sisters Jean and Mary.

I was only nine months old when my sister Mary came home from school and found our mother dead. She had suffered a massive heart attack and haemorrhage. My father and my brothers and sisters were deeply shocked. She had never complained of ill-health. She was forty-two years old.

My father felt her loss keenly. He had his own business selling court shoes for society ladies. He made them himself by hand in kid leather. Debutantes and their mothers would arrive at his door in hansom cabs, accompanied by liveried footmen and grooms, to be measured for the shoes my father made. I can recall playing with small pieces of kid leather in all sorts of magical colours, and I have always loved the smell of leather.

My father also made shoes and boots for us. I remember trying to do up my knee-length boots with a buttonhook – a silver buttonhook with a mother-of-pearl handle – and father giving me a big hug and a little present for trying.

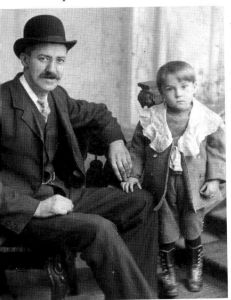

Six-year-old Eddie with my father

As his business grew, my father began to feel the strain of looking after the family, and he missed my mother so much. He started having asthmatic attacks. A housekeeper called Mary was employed to help out but she was not welcomed by the family. She slapped me because I would not call her 'mother'. This made my sisters angry. How dare she slap their baby sister!

One day my father called my brothers and sisters together. He told us that the responsibility of looking after us on his own was too much for him. He had decided to marry Mary the housekeeper. He patiently explained that it was not a love match like his marriage to our mother. It was purely for convenience, so that we could be brought up properly.

Mary did not remain long. One day she just disappeared. She took with her our mother's jewellery, amongst which was a lovely pearl necklace that my father said was to be mine if and when I reached twenty-one. It had been his wedding present to our mother. She had robbed the house of many other valuable things. William and Arthur searched for her but could trace nothing of her whereabouts. For three days and nights the front door was left open, but Mary was not to be seen or heard of again.

One by one my brothers and sisters left home. My eldest sister, Alice, got married. So did my brother Albert. For a time I went to live with Albert's in-laws – his wife's two elderly aunts.

They were kind and motherly. While living with them I had to have my tonsils and adenoids removed. The day before the operation, I was given a dose of castor oil in milk – which I promptly vomited over the clean bedclothes – but I remember my dear father visiting me. He brought me a doll and sweets, and comforted me. The next morning, as was the custom in those days, I was carried to the kitchen and laid on the scrubbed kitchen table, and there the operation was performed.

It was a horrible experience. I called out for brother Albert, but he did not come. I could not understand it. I found out later that he had left the house during the operation because he just could not bear to watch.

Albert had a brother-in-law called Colin, fourteen years old, who used to tease me and lock me up in a shed in the garden and tell me the goblins would come and eat me up. I was terrified of him. At other times he would shut me up in a dark cupboard under the stairs, saying he would leave me there to starve and no one would find me until I was a skeleton. I could tell no one of this because I was afraid he would do something dreadful to me.

Our poor father fretted for our mother. He was in and out of hospital with a chest condition. I recollect being taken to see him in hospital and being held up to kiss him. He was surrounded by cold packs.

In 1912 he died. Of a broken heart, it was said. I was four years old.

At the funeral I was carried on the shoulders of my uncle Fred. I wore a black-dotted white muslin dress with a black bow on my head and a big black sash. From that day onward I was shifted from one home to another, practically every year it seemed.

My brother Will was as good as a father to me, and gave me security. He looked like our father: tall and dark with fine long-fingered hands. He was always smartly dressed and wore grey spats over his ankles. He loved singing *Roses of Picardy* and other songs of that period.

When he was alive, our father used to gather the family together in the sitting room for a singsong on Saturdays. At that time Glory Song was popular. Gypsy Smith, the gypsy evangelist, was having a crusade and used the song as part of his mission work. The sheet music was sold in the streets. Father had bought a copy and the whole family would sit round and sing it. My brother Will tried to keep up this family tradition.

Then early in 1914, when I was just six, war broke out. William and Albert were both called up. I missed them dreadfully.

William made such a fuss of me when he came back on leave. How I looked forward to those times! Once, he brought me a pair of black lace stockings. Wearing them made me feel very grown-up.

On another leave, he announced that he had brought me a special present. It was in the front room. I had three guesses to say what it was, then I could go and find it. I said, 'A pair of shoes.' I was longing for a pair of shoes, as I had always had to wear knee-length boots. He laughed and said I was getting warm.

I hurried to the room. All I could see was a long black box with hinges. It didn't look much like shoes, and try as I might I just could not open it.

Will came in. 'Can't you get them on?'

'They will be too big,' I said, 'and must be a funny shape.'

He opened up the long black box. It was a violin.

'There you are,' he said, taking the violin out and handing it to me. 'I've arranged for you to have lessons – an hour a week.'

I found the lessons difficult, but I was so proud to walk along the street with my violin case tucked under my arm, and I began to enjoy learning to play when I started on the popular melodies of the day, songs such as In a Monastery Garden and tunes like Barcarole. I still love to hear the violin.

Every Christmas Will took me to a pantomime. One year he took me to the Lyceum to see *Cinderella*. We hadn't had time for dinner before we left so he bought some cheese, custard cream biscuits and oranges. He put his large handkerchief over my knees and cut chunks of cheese with his penknife and we ate the biscuits and oranges. Then the curtain went up and I sat enthralled. Now and then he would put his arms round me, and give me a hug. Oh, how I loved my big brother then!

After that, Will was away a long time. He had been wounded on the battlefield. His escape from death was miraculous. A bullet had hit him in the chest, but a tin of 'iron rations' which he kept in his breast pocket prevented the bullet hitting his heart. It still caused him serious injury. It ricocheted off and entered his chest wall. Several bits of shrapnel were embedded in his lungs and he had to have a series of operations. Even so, some of the shrapnel remained in one lung.

I was eventually taken to see him at Tamworth Army Hospital. He looked so strange in the blue hospital pyjamas. I loved him so much and I was afraid he would not come home again.

He did come home but he never properly recovered, and after many years of ill-health he contracted tuberculosis and died.

For a time I went to live in Norman Road, Leytonstone, with Aunt Bessie and Uncle Vernon Rashleigh and their daughters Edith and Hilda. I was very happy with them. I was still only six years old. Edith was a year older than me and Hilda was a year younger.

Uncle Vernon had a wood-carving business. We girls were allowed to play in his work-room. I loved the smell of the wood. We had great fun with the shavings, uncurling them and then dropping them on the floor or table to see what patterns or letters of the alphabet they formed. Edith was fond of collecting rose petals and making scent with them. Hilda and I felt extremely grown up whenever Edith allowed us to help by stirring the petals in the water every two or three hours.

We all went to the school round the corner in Mayville Road. Edith and Hilda got on better there than me: they were both clever little girls, especially Edith. At that time my hair was worn in two long plaits, one hanging down my front and one down my back, and it was the plait hanging down the back that got me into trouble. A boy in the seat behind me, without my knowing it, dipped the end of my plait in the inkwell and then trapped it in the hinge of his desk so that when I went to move my head it caught. I cried out because it hurt me.

The teacher – she was called Miss Gill – thought I was playing about and called me out to the front of the class. She made me write on the blackboard in big letters: I MUST NOT SHOUT IN CLASS. Then I had to kneel down and keep my eyes on the board until the lesson was over. The boy wasn't punished at all. I thought it very unfair.

Miss Gill used to think the world of Edith: it seemed that all the teachers did. After that incident with the plaits, Miss Gill told me that if I went on like this I would never be as good as my cousin.

But Miss Gill was still my favourite teacher. The pupil who had been considered the best for that week was appointed next week's monitor and was sometimes taken to stay at Miss Gill's home for the weekend. We used to be so jealous of whoever got to be monitor and I longed to be made monitor so that I too could go and stay with Miss Gill. But I never did.

In 1916 Uncle Vernon decided to take the family to Canada. He and Aunt Bessie wanted to take me with them also, but big brother William said no. He had met a young girl called Flo whom he had married when she was nineteen. Since he looked on me, and little Eddie, as his responsibility, we were both to stay with them and their own little children.

I was sad not to be able to go to Canada with my cousins. Edith wrote us a long letter describing their voyage and it was read out in assembly for the whole school to hear. Everyone thought it was marvellous.

Will and his young wife moved into the house in Norman Road. They had to take responsibility for Grandma Staerck, my father's elderly mother who had the upstairs front room. She was a formidable old lady and I was always a little in awe of her. To her dying day there was not a grey strand to be seen in her dark brown hair, and like my father she had penetrating dark eyes. Every day she had a glass of warm stout. Will would heat the poker in the fire until it was red hot then plunge it into the glass for me to take up to her. She seemed always to wear a black satin dress, a square of lace over her head, and a white shawl draped around her shoulders. I associate her with pictures of Queen Victoria, mourning for her Albert.

I was to stay with Will and Flo until I reached the age of fourteen. They had four children of their own. Flossie was the eldest, then came William, Fred and Gladys. I loved these children, though I was often kept away from school to look after them. Now I realise how difficult life must have been for Flo during this time – during the war and then through the post-war depression when Will had a hard time finding work. To help make ends meet Will began experimenting with an incubator in the shed in the back yard. He was hatching chickens' eggs. The incubator was heated with an oil lamp.

Early one morning there was a loud knocking at the door. It was the milkman. He had heard cracking glass and thought the house was being broken into. Investigating further, he found a fire raging at the back of the house. By the time he had roused us the neighbours were rallying round. When Will opened the door there were a dozen men in line passing buckets of water from hand to hand.

A cat – or something – must have got into the shed and knocked over the oil lamp. The incubator was burning and so were the day-old chicks. The fire was spreading rapidly. Someone had already called the fire brigade and when they arrived they hurried us out of the house and helped Will and Flo throw everything out of the window. It was raining by this time so all our belongings got soaked.

When the fire was well and truly out, Will and Flo looked round for their children and for Eddie and me. We were nowhere to be seen. Once again the neighbours had helped out. Each of us had been taken in by a different family to see that we were kept safe until things had quietened down. Will and Flo had quite a job finding us all again.

In place of the incubator, Will built a chicken run. He also had rabbits – white, black and fawn. They were adorable. I was so excited each time the rabbits produced litters – but desolate when one batch had to be put into a sack and drowned.

A new year started at Mayville Road school. Though Edith and Hilda were no longer there, their achievements were still used as a measure of my progress. They had been much cleverer than me – as my new class teacher made clear. He said I would have to work very hard to be anything like them.

Nevertheless I began to enjoy the lessons, especially Friday afternoons when we had a spelling bee. A long word like 'revelation' or 'cosmopolitan' would be written up on the blackboard and we had to see how many words we could make out of it. I must have had a flair for this sort of thing. I won several times. Once I was given a little Chinese doll as a prize. Proudly, I took it home and showed it to Will and Flo. But Flo said I was too old for dolls. She took it away and gave it to Flossie. I was broken-hearted.

I continued with my violin lessons, despite the teasing from my brother Eddie. He would howl and make terrible noises and grimaces as I tried to practise. He was six years older than me and we were very close. He used to sit me in a basket tied on to his skates and push me down any available slope he could find. I loved it.

Eddie had to take me to school and bring me home again. One morning I cried and cried and would not go, and clung to a bollard at the end of the street. Passers-by glared at him, thinking he was ill-treating me. He was so embarrassed. But he never took it out on me.

One day, when he came to take me home, he was wheeling his bicycle and smoking his first cigarette. He made me promise not to tell Will. There was no need to. He was green in the face by the time we arrived home, and then he vomited. Flo could tell the reason. She smelt the smoke on his clothes and found the cigarettes. They were thrown straight in the bin and he was given a big dose of castor oil and sent to bed without tea. Soon afterwards Eddie ran away and joined the Army. He was fourteen years old.

With my brother Eddie gone, I became closer to my sister Jean. To help Flo, Jean took over the responsibility of looking after me. It was she who now took me to the pantomime when Christmas came, and she saw to it that I was well clothed. She had recently gone to live with Aunt Jenny, our father's oldest sister. Aunt Jenny was godmother to several of my sisters and brothers and had been a great help to my father after mother died. Her house was in Albany Street, just by Regent's Park.

I loved my Aunt Jenny and whenever I went to stay there I never wanted to go back to Flo's. I realise now what a lot of trouble Flo took to make me look pretty. But at the time I just wanted to live with my sister Jean and Aunt Jenny.

Every night Flo used to put my long hair in curls, wound around long strips of rag. It was agony to sleep with them, but when the rags were removed I had long ringlets that were greatly admired.

Three times I tried to run away from Flo's house. I never got far. Once, after Flo had got me ready for bed, I slipped out of the house in my nightgown, curling rags in my hair, and climbed aboard a bus.

'Where are you going?' said the conductor.

'To Regent's Park, please,' I said. 'I've got no money.'

'Oh,' he said, 'so you belong to the Zoo, do you?' and promptly took my hand and handed me over to a policeman. And that was the end of that, because I was taken straight home.

Eventually I had my way. The following year, 1918, I went to stay with sister Jean and Aunt Jenny.

Number One Hundred and Thirteen Albany Street was a tall terraced house. I lived with Jean in the large attic. I was so happy to be there with her at last.

Aunt Jenny took in boarders. Jean paid her way just as the other boarders did. She had a good job in a cigar factory. From her earnings she was able to put away something each week. She intended eventually to emigrate to Canada.

The two rooms on the ground floor were let to a Dr Craig as a waiting room and a consulting room. The doctor was a large, kind Scotsman and he soon became our GP. From time to time he asked me to help him by cleaning his dispensary and dusting the bottles. In this roundabout way I was introduced to the world of medicine. He could see that I was fascinated by it all. He would sometimes ask me questions about First Aid or get me to name the bones of the body. I appreciated his interest so much.

One of the female boarders in Auntie's house was also a doctor – one of the first women to be allowed to practise medicine. I knew her as Dr Jacob, and she was on the staff of the Elizabeth Garrett Anderson Hospital for Women. Sometimes when I was in her room I would sneak a look at books on the biology of the human body, and the more I read the more I became eager to study medicine.

Aunt Jenny belonged to the Anglican church of St Paul's in Portman Square. I used to go along to the girls' bible class and soon made firm friends among them. We would spend one day a week in Regent's Park. We used to row on the lake, have a brisk walk round the park afterwards, and then picnic in the afternoon. Each of us brought something to eat or drink.

We were planning to go on holiday as a group. We discussed it in great detail: how much money we had saved, when we should go, all the different possibilities to be followed up. It was all such fun.

Sister Eva Quinnell was our bible class teacher. She was a dear woman and I came to think of her as my spiritual mother. I took to calling her 'Little Mother'. One day she announced that she was leaving to take up another post. We were so sad, but cheered up when she explained that her new post was in Eastbourne, as warden of the Christian Holiday Home. If we wrote to the current warden it might be possible for us to have our holiday when Sister Eva would be there to look after us.

We composed a letter and sent it off straight away. By return we heard that a group of up to twenty could be accommodated, full board and lodging. Now that we had a definite plan, we could focus on the details – clothes, pocket money, fares and so forth. Aunt Jenny allowed us to meet at her house to discuss everything.

We decided to pool our savings. By sharing out what we had we could all afford the holiday. In various ways we added to our savings: bazaars, raffles, bring-and-buy evenings. Aunt Jenny was a great help. She made many useful suggestions and even got a couple of her friends to judge the talent contests we held! We had auctions in Aunt Jenny's dining room. One of us would make sweets, another biscuits. I made watercolour sketches and illuminated biblical texts to display as scrolls. We all did our bit and quickly sold out of everything. With the money raised, added to what we had, we were able to afford the two weeks at Eastbourne.

We travelled there by coach and arrived one sunny Saturday in August. We were delighted with our rooms. The grounds had huge lawns. Beachy Head was a ten minute walk, with its lighthouse at the foot of the cliffs and the local beach was only five minutes down the road. Because our beloved Sister Eva was in charge we saw a great deal of her and had many opportunities for spiritual fellowship. At night we had long talks amongst ourselves – and not a few midnight feasts! Each summer for some years to come the same group of us returned to enjoy a similar holiday together.

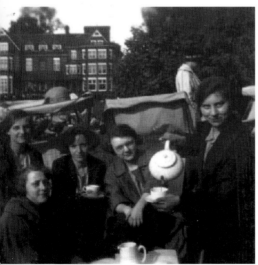

Holiday tea-party in the garden at Eastbourne, 1923

A little later in the year I was asked to accompany a young mother with two little boys to Devon on their holiday. One of the boys suffered from a severe form of eczema. He had to have a special diet and at night had to be painted with a special tar lotion and sleep between two sheets only. The mother was known to one of Aunt Jenny's friends, who was asked to try and get help. She knew I loved children, and I was pleased to oblige.

They turned out to be a delightful family. Simon, the little boy, was difficult about food and needed a great deal of coaxing to eat anything at all. At night he would get no sleep because of the pain, for as soon as he got warm the irritation would increase. In the end I suggested we all sleep in the open air on the balcony where it was cooler. Both boys loved this and felt they were having a real adventure.

I was only twelve years old but, looking back, I think this experience must have been a great help when several years later I applied for nurse training.

2

Home From Home

We know that in everything God works for good with those who love Him
Romans 8.28

When I was fourteen, Aunt Jenny took me to a conference led by Dr Marsh: the annual general meeting of the China Inland Mission. That afternoon I heard people tell how the Lord had called them to China. Missionaries who had returned spoke of the loving care and protection they had received from God in their work in the field.

In the evening there was an open air meeting in Hyde Park. I had been moved by what I had heard at the conference and during the meeting felt a stirring of my heart but did not respond until I got home that night. I went to my bedroom and knelt by my bed and asked the Lord Jesus to come into my heart.

Aunt Jenny had an Apple of Gold calendar. It was the custom at breakfast for her to tear the day's slip off and read it to us. The morning after the meeting she told me to tear off the slip and read it out. It was from Psalm 28: 'The Lord is my strength and my shield. My heart trusted in Him, and I am helped. Therefore my heart greatly rejoiceth; and with my song will I praise Him.' There followed a verse from a hymn:

Yesterday He helped me.
Today I praise His name.
For well I know tomorrow
He will help me just the same.

I turned to Aunt Jenny and said, 'I have accepted the Lord Jesus as my Saviour.'

She wanted to know when and how it had happened. I was happy to tell her, and at bible class the following Sunday I told Sister Eva about my conversion. She told me to study the bible. From that day I began to read a chapter every day.

It was while reading God's word on that first day that I realised the first step I had to take as a new-born Christian was to confess to one and all that I was God's child. In obedience to Christ I must be baptised. I was so challenged that I told Aunt Jenny that I wanted to be baptised by immersion. Since she was an Anglican she said that I should be confirmed. She would arrange for me to attend confirmation classes. But I was adamant that I wanted baptism.

After church that same Sunday she went to see Sister Eva. When she came back she said that the rector wished to see me. We both went into the rector's vestry. It was there I met Dr Stuart Holden.

He was the Home Director of the China Inland Mission. He had a great reputation as a bible scholar and was respected the world over. But he seemed a kindly man. He bade us sit down.

'I want you to speak sense to this child,' said Aunt Jenny. 'I want her to be confirmed. But she has a wild idea that she must be baptised.'

Dr Holden said to me, 'I believe you have had a call to be a missionary, haven't you?' Sister Eva must have told him this. I nodded my head. He smiled and asked Aunt Jenny to let us have a few minutes alone together.

When she had gone, Dr Holden asked me a number of questions – in particular, why I wanted to be baptised. I told him I felt I must obey Christ's word and quoted the scripture that had led to the decision. I said that I wanted to be a missionary in China. He called Aunt Jenny in and, to my relief, said to her, 'This child knows what she is doing. If we had a baptistry I would baptise her myself. But I will certainly arrange it.'

He was as good as his word. I was baptised on the twenty-sixth of April at the Marylebone Chapel Baptist Church in Marylebone Road. Afterwards the minister gave each candidate a piece of paper on which was written a text. Mine was Romans 8.28. It is a verse that has given me tremendous help and strength as the years have passed: 'And we know that all things work together for good to them that love God, to them who are called according to His purpose.' The hymn that we sang then is still one of my favourites:

> All the way my Saviour leads me.
> What have I to want beside?

Auntie Jenny was present the evening I was baptised. She had brought along a friend, Ivy Beale, who was often poorly. That night they both asked to be baptised themselves. A few short weeks later they too went through the waters. How full of joy I was!

My baptism took place on the twenty-sixth of April 1922. Exactly two years later, on the twenty-sixth of April 1924, my sister Mary was married. Jean and I were bridesmaids. Aunt Jenny made the bride's dress in white satin and decorated the bodice with pearls. She also helped Mary make the wedding cake.

Jean and I thought we looked fantastic in our dresses. We wore crêpe-de-chine with chiffon sleeves in old gold. The twenty-sixth of April was Primrose Day, so we wore a circlet of primroses in our hair and held posies of primroses. As the youngest, I had a basket of primroses which I was to sprinkle on the ground before the bride as she walked into the church.

We liked the groom, Frank Goldsmith. He was tall, with blond hair, and he played the violin divinely. He was also an artist and painted beautiful pictures in water colours and oils. The next year Mary gave birth to a daughter. They called her Margaret.

In 1927 at the age of nineteen, I began to train as a nurse. Sister Eva told me she had seen an advert in the daily paper asking for nursing probationers and suggested I applied. I did so, and was soon given a date for an interview. I was thrilled.

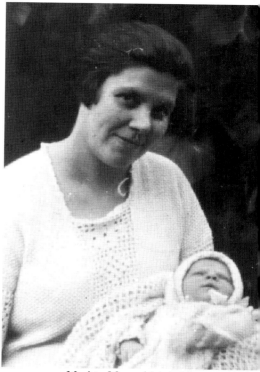

I had to have a medical check-up and be vaccinated. Aunt Jenny took me to Dr Craig for the vaccination and asked if he would give me a reference. He showed a great deal of interest in the prospect of my training to be a nurse, but as he pushed the needle in I fainted. When I came round he laughed and said, 'Now what are you going to do when you have to dress wounds and watch operations?'

I replied that God would help me because He had called me to work in China. The doctor laughed and turned to my Aunt. 'She'll do,' he said.

My sister Mary with baby Margaret, 1925

He told me I was to let him know how I was getting on. He was such an encouragement. He also said I must ask him about anything that puzzled me during my training. 'And then,' he added, 'when you pass your Finals, I'll celebrate with you.'

He kept to his word and would explain the use of various drugs and answer my many other queries. He was delighted when I eventually passed my exams and even came to the prize-giving with Aunt Jenny. But that was all in the future. For the present, I didn't even know if I would be allowed to start my training.

When I appeared before the matron for my appointment I was extremely nervous. Fortunately she was not too frightening – a tall lady with a kind face. She asked me why I wanted to train. I told her I was going to China as a missionary and nursing was important. She asked me if I liked children and old people. I replied that for some years I had lived with my eldest brother and his wife and their four children who were younger than me and that I had helped look after them. I had also cared for my Aunt when she had been ill with pneumonia. It was because of all this, I told her, that I realised I was drawn to nursing and looking after people.

'Well then,' she said, 'you may start training. The home sister will show you round and give you a list of the clothes you must bring.'

My nurse training began on the thirty-first of October. I started as a probationer at St Mary's Hospital in Islington. Aunt Jenny accompanied me with my few belongings. It was rather awe-inspiring to come to the porter's lodge and be vetted and to have to sign a huge book. The head porter told me that every time I entered or left the grounds I had to sign that book and any visitors I had would have to sign it too.

We made our way to the matron's office. She rang for her assistant matron, a large, severe-looking, full-breasted woman called Miss Anderson who escorted us to the nurses' home to meet the home sister.

The home sister first gave us a tour of the accommodation, then took us to my room. It was small and austere, containing an iron bedstead with a thin mattress and one wooden chair – not an inviting room at all.

'The bell will ring at six-fifteen every morning,' said the home sister. 'You must be washed and dressed and ready in the dining room for roll call and breakfast at 7am. By 9am you are to have tidied your rooms and made your beds before reporting to the ward sister for the day's training to begin. Don't make your beds before leaving for breakfast, because the maids strip and air them while you are eating. You'll only have to make them all over again.'

To our dismay we found this to be true!

To have my washing done I had to fill in the laundry book each Friday, put soiled clothes in the white linen bag supplied, and place it outside my door, along with the bottom sheet and one pillowcase which would be replaced with clean ones. That week's unwashed top sheet would become next week's bottom sheet. We had to supply our own towels and see to washing them ourselves.

The home sister led us to an empty room which she said was used for smoking: we were not to smoke in our rooms or the sitting room.

'Oh,' put in Aunt Jenny at once, 'my niece does not smoke and never has.'

'I expect she will get like the rest before long,' said the sister.

She took us to the sewing room and I was measured for my uniform. There was a blue cape lined with scarlet that was for use only inside the hospital grounds. A brown ankle-length cape was for outside use. To cover the head a brown crêpe-de-chine square was provided.

I was told to try on my uniform. In the morning a nurse would come to show me how to make up my cap in a butterfly pattern. It was quite a work of art and had to be learned. I was to report to matron's office at 9.30am, tidy, and wearing blue-and-red cape.

I was quite overcome by all these instructions and getting more and more nervous by the minute, but I put on the uniform and suddenly felt so proud. I was really on the way to being a proper nurse. Aunt Jenny helped me unpack and put my clothes away. Then it was time for her to leave.

We looked in the sitting room on the way out. It was nicely decorated with plenty of comfortable settees and armchairs – and two pianos.

'You will be able to keep up your piano practice,' said Aunt Jenny.

The previous year she had paid a music teacher to give me lessons for nine months. I enjoyed playing the piano so I nodded in agreement but secretly I felt I would be too nervous to practise in front of the other probationers.

I walked with her to the gate. We noted how beautiful the grounds were – rose beds in profusion dotted about the well-kept lawns. We saw that there was a tennis court marked out on the grass. Aunt Jenny said I should learn to play.

When we made our farewells she gave me a hug and a kiss. I felt absolutely desolate. I think she felt the parting also. She had been my guardian for seven years and although she was strict I knew she was fond of me – as I was of her. It was she who had led me on the Christian path. She promised that she and her friends would uphold me in prayer.

After seeing Auntie to her bus I returned to my room and had a good cry. I felt even more lonely thinking of my sister Jean. The previous year she had followed my cousins Edith and Hilda to Canada. Though she wrote regularly I missed her terribly. And now I was completely on my own. I didn't even have Aunt Jenny to comfort me.

At last I unpacked my belongings and tried to calm down. I brought to mind the text I had received at my conversion: 'He is my strength and shield.' I said a prayer, asking my heavenly Father to give me the courage I needed.

After a restless night I was awakened by the clanging of the morning bell. How I wanted to turn over and go back to sleep again. But I remembered I had a uniform to get into. I scampered to the bathroom, washed, and began to dress.

There was a knock on the door. In came the nurse who was to help me with my cap. When she was sure I was spick and span, I made my way to matron's office, where another probationer was waiting. She was a little overpowering, but friendly enough, and I soon found she was a Christian. She introduced herself as Miss Ethel Izzard and asked me if I was 'saved'. I said yes. Then she asked why I was training to be a nurse.

'The Lord has called me to China,' I told her.

'Oh, how super!' she cried. 'I'm going to Africa!'

She said we must stick together and start our missionary work here and have weekly meetings for the other nurses. 'And you know,' she said, 'we have a missionary field with all the patients, haven't we?'

I agreed and said we must pray about it. We arranged to meet daily in her room or my room for prayer and reading, and to organise a meeting. She was a strong character, confident and energetic. We

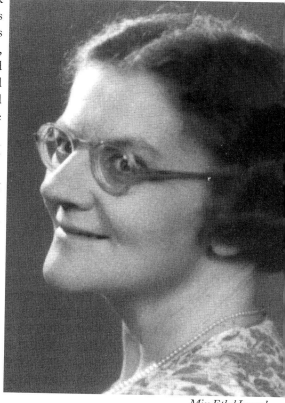

Miss Ethel Izzard

grew to enjoy each other's company and fellowship and soon became firm friends. We decided to start a Christian Nurses Fellowship at the nurses' home.

Ethel would go where angels feared to tread. She went to matron, Miss Cordell, told her of our intended venture, and asked permission to use the lounge. Miss Cordell suggested that we use the hospital chapel instead. She thought the chaplain might want to take part. We were not too keen about this. The chaplain was High Church, almost Roman Catholic, and most of the girls who would be attending the CNF meetings were free church or non-denominational. However, we agreed to try it out.

So every Wednesday evening we gathered in the chapel, which was at the very top of the hospital. We were given permission to use the organ. One of our gang was a Welsh girl called Evans. She was a keen piano-player and had never tried the organ – but she got some kind of result.

In those days we did a ninety-hour week. We were not allowed outside the gates after eight o'clock at night unless we had a pass from matron. Occasionally we were allowed an evening off – provided the ward sister could spare us and there were not too many patients. There could be as many as sixty patients per ward. But I loved my work, and so was always willing to stay later than nine. This was especially necessary during the epidemics of pneumonia when the patients were seriously ill and in need of intensive care.

These were the days before antibiotics were widely available. The following year, however, Alexander Fleming discovered penicillin. It was a dramatic breakthrough. He worked at the University of London, but he was also pathologist at St Mary's, so we heard all about what penicillin could do from the great man himself and felt privileged to be associated with him. Despite his achievements, his demeanour was humble. I believe he was also a good Christian.

We usually had one day off a week. Otherwise our hours of duty were from seven-thirty in the morning to nine o'clock at night. We had one-and-a-half hours off duty during which time we had to attend the statutory lectures that were a part of our training, as well as try to find some time to eat. The lectures were given by the consultants, and also by our sister tutor who was called Miss Nelson. She was strict and made us work hard in study. But she was thoughtful and interesting. She heard about our meetings and encouraged us. Occasionally she even came along herself – taking over from Nurse Evans at the organ.

Aunt Jenny had been told by matron on that first day that I would be allowed to sleep out one night a week, so she and her friends were looking forward to seeing me when I first arrived home in full uniform. They were all so proud of me.

Aunt Jenny's friends had all been trained as court dressmakers. Miss Waterfield and Miss Cook lived together. Miss Waterfield developed cancer of the jaw and neck and died, though she was so brave to the end. Miss Eldridge and Miss Wesley also lived together. I called each of them 'Auntie'. Then there was Miss Hurst – Auntie Milly – who came to my wedding so many years later, the only surviving member of Aunt Jenny's little group. They were so good in their support of me. They had a weekly prayer meeting and bible study. One week they asked me to give a talk about hospital life. Another week, Miss Waterfield presented me with several pairs of black woollen stockings that she had knitted. They lasted the whole of my training – and for some years later.

During the first year of my training Jean wrote in one of her letters from Canada that she was to become Mrs Mark Jones. Her husband-to-be was from Wales. She said that she and Mark would be coming home for their honeymoon so he could meet our family, and she his in North Wales. He wanted them to have a cottage in Wales for their first home.

In her letter she wished me well in my nursing and said she was proud of me. She was also proud of my brother Eddie who was now in the Royal Signals Regiment. He was doing well. He had studied hard and had become an education officer. He also played and taught various sports. He was still smoking – he was now a chain smoker – and I was very unhappy about that. He too married that year and went on to have three daughters. Over the next forty years he would be further commissioned and rise to the rank of Major. Eventually he was to die from lung cancer on his sixty-fifth birthday.

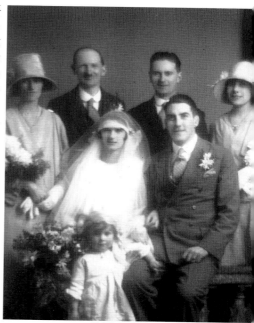
Eddie and his new wife Ivy, 1928

My cousin Edith had got a job as a florist out in Canada – she always loved plants and flowers and she loved the Canadian way of life. The following year she came back on a visit. It was her idea that we should drop in at our old school in Mayville Road. I dashed off to meet her, still dressed in my outdoor nurse's uniform – long brown cape and brown silk hat. The headmistress remembered us and seemed pleased to see us. Then we went in to see Miss Gill who was delighted that I was training to be a nurse. For once she seemed to pay more attention to me than to Edith.

'You took all the limelight,' Edith joked afterwards. 'It's because you're a nurse now and I'm just a florist.'

'Do you remember,' I replied, 'Miss Gill used to say to me, you'll never be as good as your cousin. Perhaps I've just caught up a little.'

The eleventh of March 1929 was my twenty-first birthday. In the morning I received many birthday cards from friends and relations. In the afternoon, to my great surprise and joy, Aunt Jenny visited me. She brought me a birthday cake she had made specially, just as she had done in previous years. She also brought a bag of fruit and some cucumber sandwiches to share with my nurse friends.

My present from her was really special. Aunt Jenny had given me a choice: a small radio or a tea set. I chose the tea set, and now Aunt Jenny brought it out – a beautiful tray, edged with cane, its blue base covered with glass, and to go on it a fine white bone china tea-set, decorated with bluebirds. In addition, there was a big tablecloth, a tea cosy and a serviette – all hand-embroidered with matching bluebirds by my aunt.

I was thrilled. When I showed the nurses they said, 'We must christen them.' They suggested we had a party at the CNF meeting to be held the following day.

The next evening I made some tea in the china teapot and carried the tea set down to the sitting room on the beautiful tray. I prayed all would go well. We had arranged a special speaker – Miss Eva Quinnell – my old bible class leader whom I called 'Little Mother'. She was now Deaconess at St Paul's Church, Portman Square. She had already done so much for me, guiding me to apply for nursing and helping me in my spiritual life. I was delighted she was able to be at my twenty-first birthday party as well.

As I brought in my precious china, Nurse Evans and Ethel Izzard appeared with plates of cream buns, shortbread slices and buttered scones. They had popped to the confectioners that afternoon. Birthday cake and cucumber sandwiches were added to the feast, everyone sang 'Happy Birthday', and we tucked in. Then it was time for the meeting. Miss Quinnell gave her testimony. We were deeply moved. Eventually, two of our group went to the mission field. A girl called Florence took up a mission to Persia and Ethel ended up – not in Africa as she had intended, but in China – with the China Missionary Society.

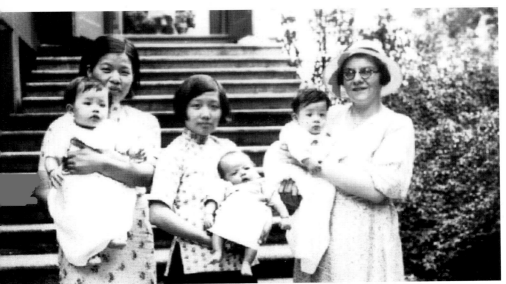

Nurse Izzard on the mission field

3

The Visiting Angel

Do not neglect to show hospitality to strangers,
for thereby some have entertained angels unawares
Hebrews 13.2

Would there be buns for tea? That was the question in our minds on the days a CNF meeting was held. On those days one of the girls would go to the confectioners at Archway Corner and see if there were any leftover buns to be had at a reduced price. If there were, we would serve them up with a cup of tea after the meeting.

For one of our meetings we invited a Mrs Dagmar André to speak. She was the wife of the wealthy businessman Paul André, associate of racing driver Sir Malcolm Campbell. What was more important for us was that Mrs André was also a prominent Christian worker. She was extremely active in promoting the Strangers' Rest Mission and was going to tell us about its work in the Docklands.

It happened to be my turn to get the buns. I had on my long brown cape. Returning from Archway Corner, buns safely in my bag, I was stepping down from the tram when a car rushed past. It caught my cape and I was flung on to the bonnet. The car did not stop and I was carried along with it.

I managed to hold on by grabbing one of the large lamps that cars had in those days. The car raced up the Archway with me holding on for dear life. I don't know if the driver was aware of his extra passenger, but plenty of people on the street saw it. They stared and pointed as I went past.

Fortunately there was a compulsory stop outside the hospital. The car came to a halt and I clambered off. The driver didn't seem to notice me. Either that or he was ignoring me on purpose. As the car drove off I walked unsteadily towards the hospital gates. Amazingly, I was still clutching my bag with its precious store of buns.

The porter saw me coming up the drive and called out, 'Nurse Staerck, you've got a visitor.'

'Oh, have I?' I said meekly. I was still in a daze.

'I told her to go up to the nurses' home and wait there for you.'

I thanked him and started walking in that direction. Everything had an air of unreality about it. I was at one remove from myself.

'She's in a posh car,' he called after me.

As I approached the Nurses' Home, I saw a sleek car with wide running boards. A handsome lady stood by it. Her hair was golden. She looked like an angel. While I was still some way off she introduced herself in a strong voice as Mrs André.

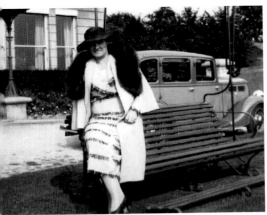

Mrs Dagmar André and her sleek car

'I've come to take the meeting,' she said. 'You must be Mina Staerck.'

As I came closer she could see that all was not well. 'What's the matter with you? You look terrible. Have you had a shock?'

Mrs André had piercing blue eyes and a fine peaches-and-cream complexion. She seemed kind enough in a fierce sort of way. I told her about the incident with the car.

'Somebody ought to know,' she said at once. 'Shall I tell the matron?'

'No,' I said. 'Don't tell the matron. I might get into trouble.' I started to tremble.

'You'd better sit down,' she said and motioned to one of the running boards of her car. I was shivering all over.

That evening Ethel Izzard led the meeting and introduced our guest speaker. Mrs André told the story of her conversion.

She spoke frankly and directly. She started by telling us that she could not have children. This had caused her marriage to founder and she was now estranged from her husband. She had wanted to adopt a child. She thought it might help heal the rift in her marriage but she also felt that by adopting a child she would be using her privileged position in some positive way.

Dr F B Meyer ran a celebrated orphanage. She went along to see him. He advised her against adopting a child. 'That would be helping just one person,' he said. 'But, you know, there is work you can do where you can help many people.'

He spoke to her of a mission in the East End called the Strangers' Rest and arranged a meeting with Miss Cleaver, the deaconess of the mission. Mrs André described how at once she hopped into her sports car and drove down to see Miss Cleaver. She was made welcome. Miss Cleaver showed her around and explained why the mission was called the Strangers' Rest. It was for the many sailors from all parts of the world who day by day landed at the docks of London. In a strange and perhaps hostile city the mission provided food, a place to stay, and the opportunity to meet others.

'There's just one thing I want to know,' said Miss Cleaver over a cup of tea. 'How do you stand spiritually?'

Mrs André did not know quite what to say. Then Miss Cleaver brought out a little book called *Safety, Certainty and Assurance*. It was a tract with the subtitle The Way of Salvation.

'I want you to read this as soon as you get home. Read it and consider it carefully. Then you'll be able to tell me where you stand.'

Mrs André took the booklet and set off home in her sports car. She was perplexed but intrigued, so she pulled into a by-way and started to read the tract there and then. It described the spiritual life in terms of a railway journey. When you board the train, you are full of faith that you will arrive safely at your destination. You place your trust in the driver of the train. God oversees our lifetime journey. By placing your life in the hands of the Lord, you receive His certainty and assurance. As soon as she had finished the booklet Mrs André turned her car around and drove straight back to the mission.

'I know where I stand,' she said to Miss Cleaver. 'I'm seeking. I want to be safe, certain and sure.'

At Miss Cleaver's prompting they knelt down and prayed. That was when Mrs André gave herself to the Lord. From that time onwards the mission became the most important thing in her life. She poured everything into it – and that included her husband's money. Even though they were estranged, she always managed to wheedle something out of him, and often it was a sizeable amount.

Mrs André's talk went down exceptionally well. At the end, she gave out copies of *Safety, Certainty and Assurance* to each nurse, along with a little book she had written called *Ransomed,* which was the story she had just told – the story of her conversion.

After the meeting, in view of the incident with the car, Ethel saw to it that I got to bed straight away. Despite my protestations, Mrs André had insisted on telling the home sister about what had happened. The home sister was Irish and had a lisp. She came to see how I was.

'Now, Mith Thtaerck. You mutht prothecute.'

I told her I did not believe in prosecutions.

'Oh, you mutht,' she replied. 'Theeth fartht driverth might kill thombody.'

I said it was up to the Lord to avenge His elect. I would leave it to Him.

'You could have been killed,' agreed the doctor the next day, after I had described what had happened. 'It's a wonder your back wasn't broken.'

Fortunately, he could find no sign of any physical injury. But he asked to see me again in two weeks' time, just to make sure.

When I got back to the nurses' home, a basket of Parma violets had arrived for me. They were accompanied by a little note.

> I hope you are better. Look forward to seeing you at 85 Finchley Road whenever you like. Mrs André.

I soon took her up on her invitation. I felt drawn to her. She had been so kind and caring to me at our first meeting – just like a visiting angel.

Eighty-five Finchley Road seemed to me to be a mansion. She lived there in some luxury, with a maid to look after her and everything she could possibly want provided for her by her husband. Everything, that is, except a child of her own. I discovered she was Swedish. That accounted for the blue eyes and golden hair. Her maiden name was Abrahamsson.

During 1930 we took our Preliminary Examination, set by the General Nursing Council, and the Hospital Junior Examination. By the grace of God I passed both, coming top in the Junior exam. Miss Nelson, our tutor, was delighted at our

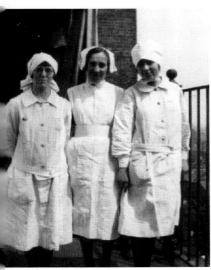

Life on the top floor

success. She was soon to be leaving the hospital and we were sad because she had helped us so much. But that day we all celebrated.

For those probationers who had passed the exam it was a happy day when we were told to get laundry baskets and put our belongings into them, ready for a porter to transport them to the new nurses' home.

We were to live on the top floor of the newly built home. In each room was a large built-in wardrobe, where we could store our cases and precious belongings.

We also had a wash-basin in the room – which was a real luxury. The bathrooms were modern and there were many of them. No more queuing for baths – and always plenty of hot water! Our beds were wooden with colourful bedspreads and – a real luxury – interior-sprung mattresses. There was a fire escape where we would often sit. From the top steps we had a fine view across North London.

My tea set was used regularly. At the end of the month on pay days we would have cream buns to go with our tea – most enjoyable, although not too good for our figures! But in those days we did not care.

Our pay was £18 per year, out of which we had to pay for our examinations. The fees made a big hole in our pay packets. But we were happy and enjoyed our nursing and training in spite of the long hours. It was nursing with procedures that are now no longer undertaken: hot and cold packs, ice compresses, four-hourly back treatments for every patients, bed baths, nursing patients with rheumatism between blankets, all this was the order of the day – and extremely hard work.

The first day I spent on the ward I will never forget. I was sent to the Children's Ward, a long room with fifteen beds to each side. When I presented myself for duty, only the staff nurse was in attendance. Most of the other nurses were at a prize-giving ceremony. I was taken round the ward, shown the sluice and a stock of rubber sheets. There were two to each bed – a long one over the mattress, then a bottom and top sheet, a narrow mackintosh for use under a drawer-sheet, two blankets and counterpane, then a bright red blanket folded at the bottom of the bed.

It was then my job to make tea for the children. There was bread and butter and jam for sandwiches. That first day the ward maid was to show me how. But first it was time for me to eat. Off I went to the large dining room at the other end of the hospital.

It was the custom to wait at the door until a senior nurse came. Then we had to open the door for her. On no account were we to go into the dining room first. We sat at an enormously long table. The home sister or assistant matron would sit at the head, serving the food. Dishes of vegetables were passed down the table and each nurse helped herself. We were lucky if there was any food left by the time the dish reached those of us at the bottom of the table.

There were large jugs of milk. We were encouraged to drink as much milk as we wished. The extra nourishment, we were told, would be good for us during our training. The food was quite good, and for sweet it seemed there was always rice pudding: thick and creamy and most enjoyable. We had to ask to be excused by the home sister or assistant matron if we wanted to leave the table, and if any of the seniors left before us, a junior had to get up and open the door for her. If you were unlucky enough to have a seat near the door, you would be up and down like a jack-in-the-box.

Those days during the training years were simple, happy times; and I must put in a word about my ward sister, Miss Ida Johns. She taught me so much and was so considerate to me – and she probably helped saved my life when I fell ill the following year.

As my training and the practical nursing continued, I found I was spending more and more time with Dagmar André. I enjoyed my visits to Finchley Road and she would love me to accompany her on all the visits she made. There was no doubt about it, Mrs André and I had taken to each other in a big way.

She began to look upon me as a kind of adopted daughter. She called me her 'child', and I fell into calling her 'Auntie'. Though she had many visitors and invited all sorts of people to stay, I would be the only one she allowed in her house whenever I liked. She set aside a room for me. Soon I was spending much of my time there.

She had a cottage on the border of Surrey, in Sutton near Cheam. It was about three hundred years old and in a beautiful woodland setting. She loved inviting people to stay there: people from the Strangers' Rest Mission, or nurses from the various hospitals with which she was involved. A housekeeper was in permanent residence there to look after the place.

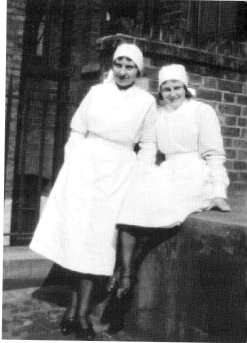

Often I went with her into the East End to help her with her work. She would arrange to pick up the family of one of the seamen connected with the mission. She would take them back to her cottage, where they stayed until their own home had been completely cleaned through and redecorated. They returned to find gleaming china, a meal on the table and a fire burning in the grate.

She did this time and time again and helped so many people when they were in difficulties. The number of lives she touched and the comfort she bestowed is beyond knowing. I soon realised that the first impression I had of her – that day she came to speak to us – was well founded. She really was a visiting angel.

* * *

On probation at St Mary's Islington, 1930

1931 was the year we were to sit our major exams: the Hospital Senior and the Final State Examination. While studying for them, I was also taking a Bible study correspondence course, run from the China Inland Mission. It touched on the fundamental basics of one's belief and there were some deep-searching questions to answer. The papers had to be sent to a Mr Hogben at CIM House. In addition to all this there was a prayer meeting every Wednesday held at the CIM headquarters in Stoke Newington. I managed to get to these whenever I was off duty.

Perhaps I worked a little too hard during those months because I had several attacks of sub-acute rheumatism. My ankles would suddenly swell, or my knees would blow up and be terribly painful. Then suddenly I contracted rheumatic fever and ran an alarmingly high temperature.

I was nursed in a side ward under Sister Johns' personal care. She was the perfect nurse. I was not allowed to move from my bed. I lay between heavy blankets to make me sweat and I was given a powerful diuretic to encourage excess fluid to leave my body. Fluid intake was restricted to protect my kidneys. After the worst was over, I made a speedy recovery. I had been extremely ill, but thanks to Sister's expert attention, I was able once again to concentrate on preparing for the exams.

Ethel Izzard and I revised together every evening. We also prayed about it together. By the time the day of the big exams was upon us, we were all extremely apprehensive. The exams were in two parts: Written and Practical. We had to go to St Mary's Hospital in Paddington for both. On the morning of the Written, I asked the Lord for help and I turned to my Bible and Daily Light and read for that day: 'The Lord is with you and will never forsake you. Be of good courage and trust in Him.' What better assurance could I have than that? I was comforted and cast all my anxiety upon Him.

When we set off, I found the other girls were fretful.

'Aren't you worried?' Nurse Evans asked me.

I had been, I said, but now I committed it all to the Lord. I would leave worrying to Him.

At St Mary's Paddington we were received by the matron, Miss Milne. She led us to the dining room where coffee and biscuits were served to us. She put us at our ease and wished us well. Then the assistant matron took us over to the school. She gave us some good advice: not to rush through the questions, and to answer first the one we felt we could do the best and then the one we felt we could do second best and so on. The examiners marking the scripts would thus from the beginning be given a good impression which would influence them in the following questions. This advice I have never forgotten. When I became a tutor of nurses myself, I made sure I passed it on to my students.

We took our seats and the senior tutor told us to look at the script on our desks and to check that the number there was the same as the one on our entrance card. She explained that she would call out the time and would warn us when we were nearing the end of the session. She told us we were not to speak, and to raise our hand if we needed more paper. She hoped we had coloured pencils with us, because drawings – if reasonably well executed – brought extra marks.

'There should be no rubbing out or smudges,' she said, adding that no one would be allowed to leave the room during the exam and we must bear that in mind.

Ethel Izzard immediately put up her hand. 'Excuse me, sister. Supposing we want to go to the toilet?'

'You will still not be allowed to leave the room,' answered the sister. 'You must control yourselves until the exam is finished and all scripts handed in. Now,' she continued, 'read carefully each question before attempting it. And good luck.'

The schoolroom was large and airy. You could hear the traffic on the road passing the hospital and the trains shunting to and from Paddington Station. I thought at first that all that noise would affect my concentration, but it did not and I was reminded again of the word of the Lord given me that morning and was comforted.

At last the bell rang and sister said, 'Put down your pens at once. Close your scripts. Be sure your name and number are clearly displayed. Take a big breath, the exam is over. You may leave now – quietly please. Oh, one thing more – the results will not be posted for eight to ten weeks. However, do not worry in the meantime, for if you have done the best you can, you will no doubt be surprised at the result. I hope it will be a happy one. Goodbye to you all.'

The first thing we all did was rush to the cloakroom. What relief! Then we quizzed each other about the difficulty – or otherwise – of the paper, what questions had been answered and how we thought we had fared. The amazing thing was that I had really enjoyed it. So had Ethel Izzard. But she was naturally clever. There was no danger of her failing the exam.

The matron of our hospital had left word at the gate that she wished to see us when we returned. We all trooped to her office. She asked how we had got on. We showed her the question paper. She read through the questions and pronounced them fair.

'Don't get worrying about what you might have written,' she said. 'You cannot do anything about it now. When we get the results, they will be put on the notice board in the dining room. Now get along for your meal. You must be ready for it.'

That afternoon one of the girls suggested a visit to Lyons Corner House in Leicester Square. We thought it a great idea, but could we afford it? The Corner House was a favourite evening outing for us, but we usually could afford it only on pay day. Then we might even treat ourselves to a Knickerbocker Glory, feeling very flush because we had a few more pennies in our purse. But pay day was still two weeks off. We decided to see what money we had and pool it. After careful calculation it seemed that between us there was just about enough for a roll and butter each, and a pot of tea.

We set off at around six-thirty. We decided to save the bus fare and walk. It took us about an hour, but we enjoyed every minute. It was early summer, the air was fresh, the skies were blue – and we had just finished our exams!

On arriving at the Corner House, we made our way to the floor where the palm court orchestra was playing. Our roll and butter and tea lasted us the whole evening as we sat there enjoying the music – the piano, violin, and cello. And the money saved by not using the bus meant our funds could stretch to a shared ice cream. Then there was the long, lovely walk home, back to St Mary's Islington.

It might be thought this was a poor way to celebrate our relief that the exams were over, but for us it was a great treat. That night the air was cool and crisp, and exhilarating.

When we reached home we had a praise meeting for the help we felt the Lord had given and for Miss Milne, the matron of St Mary's Paddington, who had been so encouraging. Many years later, Miss Milne and I would meet again in quite different circumstances. But more of that in a later chapter.

Because we had had such an enjoyable evening, we decided to save up for another outing to Lyons when the results came out, and to indulge ourselves in a salad supper at the Salad Bowl. As things turned out, Ethel Izzard topped the exam that year. That was no surprise to anyone. But to my amazement, I managed to come second.

My dear sister Jean had sent me a few dollars to celebrate when I knew the results. With her usual faith in me, she said she knew they would be worth celebrating. I told the girls that I was adding this money to our pool of funds to spend at Lyons. We were able to celebrate in style.

There was a further bonus to doing well in the exams. Ethel and I had the opportunity to choose between midwifery training at St Leonard's Hospital, Hoxton – together with an honorarium of £10 for the year – or a course in massage and physiotherapy at St Mary's. Matron asked us what we would choose. Ethel was in no doubt. She told the matron that she wanted to do midwifery because, she said, she was going to China as a missionary.

'Since Miss Izzard has chosen midwifery,' said the matron, 'will you be choosing the physiotherapy, my dear?'

'Oh no, matron,' I answered, 'I'm going to be a missionary too. The midwifery would be much more useful to me.'

'Well,' she said, 'I'll see that you are included in the midwife training course. But I'll also ask you to attend the physiotherapy school here every Saturday morning. They need a nurse to help them out, and you'll learn a lot by watching.'

I certainly did.

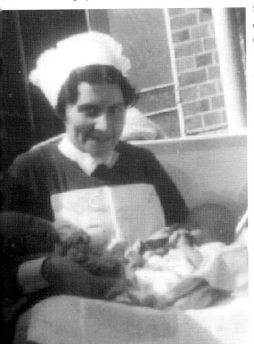

My first delivery at St Leonard's, Hoxton

4

My First Unhappy Love

I sought him whom my soul loves; I sought him, but I found him not
Song of Solomon 3.1

The China Inland Mission correspondence course bore fruit. In 1932 I won a place at their Lady Candidates Missionary Training College in Highbury. The warden was Miss Eltham, a spirited lady who had spent years in China herself. The girls were from all parts of the country and from all backgrounds. About thirty of us lived in the college. Our time was divided into theory and practical work. There were three terms to the year. Between terms we were encouraged to find some means of work to help pay for our expenses and our fares to China.

I heard there was need of a relief sister at the Capel Hanbury Hospital which was part of a Dr Barnardo's boys home near Woodford Bridge in Essex. I had been feeling that to become effective as a missionary I would need a wider range of nursing experience. The Barnardo's job seemed a godsend. I sat down at once to write the letter of application.

To my alarm I discovered I had no stamp. At that time stamps were three ha'pence each. With barely enough money to last to the end of term, I could not think how I should be able to get a stamp and send the letter off: the rules of conduct at the college were strict, and it was made quite clear that we were not allowed to make known our need of money – not even by praying aloud for it. Nevertheless, I prayed to the Lord then and there, in the privacy of my own room, for Him somehow to grant me the means of sending my letter.

One of the girls, Lilly, suffered from migraine, and that day – it was a Wednesday – she was feeling poorly. The weather was terrible. It was pouring with rain. In the afternoon I took her up a cup of tea. I asked if she would be going to the prayer meeting at CIM headquarters.

'Oh no,' said Lilly, 'I couldn't face it. My head's terrible.'

I drew the curtains and put her tea by the bed.

'Well look, this'll help you,' I said. 'And if you can manage it, I'll walk with you to the meeting. It's only ten minutes away.'

I left her to have a sleep and about an hour later I went up to see her again. She seemed a little better. 'Come on, the walk will do you good,' I said. 'It will clear your head.'

She got dressed and we set off for the meeting. The road outside was filled with puddles from the heavy showers. Looking down to avoid stepping in one, I suddenly noticed something glinting in the dirt. It was a sixpence. I picked it up at once. 'Oh!' I exclaimed, 'This is an answer to prayer,' and I told Lilly about the letter I had written and the stamp I needed. 'And now here's sixpence. I can get four stamps now.'

That was an experience I never forgot. If I learned anything at that time it was that prayer will be answered if we have faith to believe. The Lord has said in His Word, 'If you ask, I will do.' I had asked Him to supply my need and if there was any doubt that he wanted me to take up this post at Barnardo's, then here was the answer. I sent the letter off the following morning, enclosing a stamped addressed envelope, and soon received a reply – an invitation to work at the Barnardo hospital for one month.

Thomas John Barnardo was Irish, born in Dublin. He was a student at the Great London Hospital and had come into contact with fellow student Hudson Taylor, the founder of our CIM. They became great friends, and Barnardo was almost won over to go to China as a missionary himself. But he was beginning his care for the waifs and strays in the capital, and all the homeless children, and this demanding and needful work gradually became his full-time mission. He had no money, but he did have faith in the Lord. He simply set himself the task of caring for orphans and the work grew. The Lord provided for it and made it possible.

Within a few weeks I arrived to work at the Boys' Garden City. The Capel Hanbury Hospital had about a hundred beds. There was a nurses' home, a surgical ward and a well-equipped theatre. The matron was getting on – Miss Phillips was her name – but she was glad to see me and gave me a great welcome. I found I enjoyed every minute of the work and I loved working with the children.

When it was getting close to the end of the month, I was almost sorry to think I would have to leave the Boys' Garden City, even though I would be returning to the CIM college. The few weeks had been a valuable time of training for me. A few days before I was to leave, Miss Phillips came to me.

'You know, nurse,' she said, 'I shall be retiring within the next few years, and I should be so happy to think that you could be in charge, that you could take over from me.'

'Oh, I couldn't do that,' I said, though of course I was flattered. 'I'm going to China and I must continue with my training. Besides, I haven't had the experience to be a matron. Yes, I'm an SRN and a midwife – and those qualifications will be necessary for China – but I couldn't take over a matron's post.'

'Think about it,' she persisted, 'and pray about it. I'm praying about it too. But remember I would love you to take over one day. You have the makings of a matron.'

'If it's the Lord's will,' I said, 'He'll show me the way.'

'Yes, indeed,' she replied. 'There are children in all parts of the world in need of loving care. But get

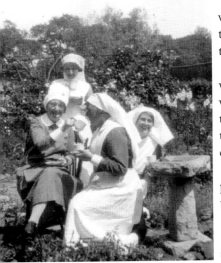

Matron Phillips and Sisters, 1932

some experience in administration,' she added. 'That would be a real help for you in China, when you eventually get there.'

With this unexpected idea in mind, I left the Boys' Garden City and returned to the college. I began to pray that if the Lord wanted me to be a matron, oh let it be a matron in China, please. And it was not long after returning to the CIM college for the next term that I was at last accepted by the Sailing Council for missionary work in the field. I had to go for a routine medical and was examined by a Dr Bragg.

A few weeks later they informed me that my sailing expenses had come through. This was the final hurdle. I was sure that nothing now could prevent me from following in Hudson Taylor's footsteps and becoming a missionary in China. Since my conversion I had read all the books I could get about China. *The Life of Hudson Taylor* was one of them. Hudson Taylor was the first missionary to China. He founded the China Inland Mission. I was a great admirer of his.

A day or two later I was working in the garden when Miss Eltham came across to me. She said, 'Mina, I've got some news for you.'

I was thrilled. I thought she was going to tell me what day I was sailing. But instead she said, 'I'm sorry, dear. I'm afraid you won't be going to China after all. Your medical wasn't good. There was something in your blood and you've got a little heart murmur there somewhere. The counsellors said that if you did go to China you wouldn't last six months. They couldn't pass you, dear. I'm so sorry.'

She knew it would be a great shock to me, and a great sadness. I had everything ready. I had drawn up lists of things to get and my trunks were already packed ready to be sent off to await my arrival. I could not understand this setback. My call to China had been so real. Yet I had to face the fact that for whatever reason the Lord had closed the door.

I unloaded all my disappointment on Sister Eva. She was upset for me and immediately got me an appointment with Dr Stuart Holden, the home director of the mission who had made it possible for me to be baptised all those years ago. When I went to talk to him, he said to me, 'Mina, I think the Lord has a special work for you to do, a work that is just beginning. I have someone here who will tell you all about it.'

He called in a young man of about thirty and introduced him as Dr Douglas Johnson, the General Secretary of the Intervarsity Fellowship. At Dr Holden's prompting, Dr Johnson told me there was a new mission starting up in London. It was called the Lansdowne Place Medical Mission. He was to be its first doctor. He would be delighted if I joined him as its first nurse. 'There's a great need out there' he said. 'We'll meet it together.'

I was enthused by his description of the work to be done. He spoke so passionately about it and he cleverly included me in his vision of what could be done. He arranged to take me round to see the mission and I gladly agreed.

Dr Holden saw that we were both on the same wavelength. He put his arms around both of us and said, 'The Lord has planned that you two should work together. I'm sure of this. The mission will be a great venture. It's a challenge to you both.'

On the appointed day Douglas Johnson showed me around the mission building. It was an old converted warehouse in Law Street, Borough, which was then a terribly poor area. This was in the days before the NHS when not everyone, certainly not many of the people in this area, could get access to adequate medical treatment.

There was a waiting room where they held services each day, and a consulting room, a small treatment room and a dispensary, all on the same floor. On the roof of the warehouse was the flat that I would occupy: one small living room, a little kitchen and a WC. The bath was in the kitchen. It had a wooden top that served as the kitchen table. From the room you could step out of a door on to a concrete ledge, a kind of balcony.

After showing me around, he welcomed me and reiterated his hopes for the mission and our part in it. 'We'll make a good team,' he said.

And we did. I worked there for almost three years. It was hard work, but I loved it. I earned twenty-seven shillings a week, out of which I had to pay for everything apart from accommodation. It didn't go far. At night, after we saw the patients, we would write notes and discuss the day's work. Then there would be the visits to the houses round about.

I had always been anaemic, and for some time had been suffering occasional abdominal pains. One night, not long after I joined the mission, I was exchanging notes in the consulting room with Dr Johnson when suddenly I felt faint and collapsed. He put my head between my knees and asked the dispenser to get me some sal volatile. He lifted me on to the consulting couch and listened to my heart. He suspected it might be a grumbling appendix, but he also thought my general physical condition was not good.

'You're not eating enough,' he said. 'What have you had today?'

At the time I was trying to do what Hudson Taylor did. He lived on just two little rolls and a bit of fish a day. Dr Johnson told me I must eat more than that. In the following days and weeks he saw to it that I did.

As we worked together over those two years we became close and grew extremely fond of each other. There was not much time for socialising, for there was so much work to be done, but on Sundays we would walk to church together. He got into the habit of calling on me in the evenings, just to see if I was all right. Our friendship deepened.

I knew I was falling in love with him and I thought he was feeling the same, though he always said he wanted our friendship to remain 'platonic'. His actions belied his words, however, and I found it confusing. He would often scribble affectionate notes to me. If he was away at a conference he would write love letters to me and conclude by writing, 'Burn this!' He treated me as if we were almost engaged. The evenings he came to visit me he would kiss me and fondle me. Sometimes he would dash in and say, 'I couldn't get here quick enough.'

We would discuss what the future held for us both. We imagined running our own mission together. In many ways things seemed so right between us. Auntie Dagmar took to him straight away. She first met him when she came to bring me some china for the flat. I remember she also brought along two cooked chickens, one for me and one for the doctor she had heard so much about.

Auntie had moved to a house in St John's Wood by that time. Sometimes when I went to stay with her she invited him to stay too. She would get me to wear one of her own beautiful dressing gowns around the house. When she was out of the room he would sit beside me on the sofa and make love to me. I was scared stiff she would come in and see us. The pretence that what we had was merely 'platonic' had long since been given up. It was, though, important for him that other people should not find out. I understood that he did not want the mission people to know. But it saddened me that he did not want his parents to know about us either.

He did warn me once. 'You know,' he said, 'this can't come to anything. I can't marry you. I mustn't. My parents sacrificed a lot for me to go to Cambridge. I have to support them.'

I felt it was wrong for him to be able to say this and yet continue to act in the way he did towards me. He was certainly very much in love with me, and I was by this time besotted with him. It was absolutely the first time I had ever been in love with anybody and the feelings were incredibly intense.

That summer – it was 1935 – I was on holiday again at Eastbourne. While I was there, I got a pain in my stomach which did not go away. It grew worse during the night and I couldn't sleep. Ethel Izzard alerted Sister Eva, our warden. 'Little Mother' was worried about my condition and rang Douglas Johnson. He guessed it was my appendix again and said he would come in the morning to take me to a nursing home in Harley Street where he sometimes worked. The doctor there was a homeopath, as well as a practitioner of conventional medicine. His name was Chave-Cox.

Douglas arrived by train and had a taxi waiting to take us back to the station. Sister Eva was reluctant to let me go but Douglas said he would ring and tell her how I was as soon as we got to our destination. The train was the Pullman Express. He had booked us into a first class compartment and we had breakfast in the dining car. I was unaccustomed to such luxury. It was my first time on a Pullman, and I had never travelled first class before.

As we ate breakfast, he sat beside me and kept hugging me. We took a taxi to the nursing home where I was introduced to Dr Chave-Cox and the distinguished surgeon who was to operate on me, Mr Anthony Raven. He was later to be knighted, but not I think for his work on me – though it was to prove a challenging operation.

When Mr Raven examined me, he decided to operate straightaway. There would be no difficulty about how I was to meet the bill for surgery. As a favour to Douglas it was understood that he would waive his usual fee. He would even allow me free use of his Harley Street nursing home to recuperate. Douglas put on gown and mask and stayed with me as I was prepared for surgery and given the anaesthetic.

The day after the operation, in came Douglas with a large bunch of flowers.

'Here's your wreath,' he said. He had a peculiar sense of humour. 'I've got the flowers all ready for your funeral.'

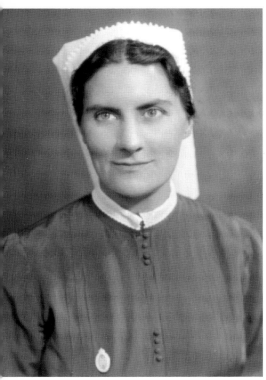

Mina Staerck, SRN, 1933

'I do feel terrible,' I said. 'I'm so sore.'

He sat on the side of the bed. 'I saw it all,' he said. 'I couldn't bear it when Raven got his knife out and started cutting into you, into your lovely flesh.'

Then he told me what they had found. It had been a difficult operation. They thought they would be dealing with a simple septic appendix, half an inch of inflamed tissue that could be just snipped out. When they opened me up they discovered that my appendix had grown to a length of nine-and-a-half inches. It had wound itself round the intestine. That was the cause of the abdominal pains. I was left with a long, nasty scar.

Douglas brought me a book to read: *Pilgrim's Progress* by John Bunyan. I had not read it before. We took it in turns to read it aloud to each other. From then on he called me 'Christiana'. He was a rare one for giving people nicknames. I called him 'Great Heart'.

I was going to have to convalesce at the nursing home for a week or so. Douglas called in each day to see me. He also wrote to me daily. The letters were beautiful, expressing all that he felt for me. He wrote well and it was like reading poetry. Each letter came with strict instructions not to keep it. 'Burn this!' became the inevitable and rather romantic postscript.

To give myself something to do while I was recuperating, I asked Douglas to buy me wool and needles from the Scottish Wool Shop, which was close by. I had never knitted anything before – I had always been much too busy – but by the time I was ready to leave I had managed to knit him a rather peculiar-looking pair of socks.

After I left the nursing home I went to stay at Auntie's, but it was not long before I was back in the same nursing home to have my tonsils out. The operation I had endured on the kitchen table all those years ago had not entirely rooted out the problem, according to Dr Chave-Cox, and he suggested having another go.

It all meant that I had to be away from the mission for some considerable time. A few days after my second operation the phone rang. Auntie's maid brought the phone to me. It was Douglas. 'Where are you?' I said.

'Liverpool Street Station. I want to take you out for the day. Got to go to Cambridge. You know, it would do you good to have a day out.'

'It's Douglas,' I said to Auntie. 'He wants to take me to Cambridge.'

'You're not well enough,' she said.

'Well, he said it would be all right, and he's the doctor.'

She wasn't happy about it, but eventually she agreed that I should at least meet him at the station. When I got there, he was absolutely determined that I should accompany him to Cambridge.

'Look, I've got an appointment with Sutton Seed Merchants. You can look round while I'm with them and then we'll meet for tea. Have you ever been to Cambridge?'

'No.'

'It's beautiful. Besides, I've already got the tickets. The seats are booked. We must go. You'll love it.'

We arrived in Cambridge and went to a nearby restaurant for coffee. He was right. It was a beautiful city and I enjoyed so much being with him. We arranged to rendezvous at the café after his meeting was over.

'Order tea at four o'clock,' he said. 'That will give us half an hour together before we have to catch the train.'

I agreed. I was looking forward to the idea of exploring the city and then meeting up with him again. I had been cooped up indoors for so long. This was a great adventure. As we left the café, he told me there was an unusual little church he wanted to show me. 'It's called the Round Church,' he said. As we went in he put his arm round me and hugged me. He said how much he loved me. Inside the church we stood arm in arm.

'Do you remember,' he said, 'I went to that conference the other week?'

'Oh, yes. How did it go?'

'Very well,' he said. 'In fact, I met a girl there. A teacher. I'm going to marry her.'

I went numb. 'You can't mean this,' I said.

'It's the best way,' he said. 'She's of a missionary family. My parents would think it right.'

He didn't seem in the least upset by what he was telling me, and when he saw how deeply upset I was he told me not to be silly. 'Believe me, it's for the best,' he said, and he gave me a peck on the cheek and left me, just like that, in the foyer of the church.

I sat down in a pew. I felt at one remove from everything. I didn't know what to do. I broke my heart, sitting there. I just couldn't understand it. First China and now this. I cried and cried.

Somehow, I made my way to the café for the arranged time and ordered tea. When he arrived he acted as if everything was the same between us. He was telling me how well the meeting had gone. I started to cry.

'Don't be foolish,' he said gently. 'Don't cry. I still love you.'

'You can't do,' I said. His tone was so unemotional. He acted as if everything could continue as it had done. I couldn't bear to prolong my agony a moment longer. 'I want to go back,' I told him.

When we got to Liverpool Street station, I was in such a state that he put me in a taxi, paid the driver and told him to be sure when he dropped me off at Eighty-five Finchley Road to ring the bell for me.

The maid opened the door. 'Hello, Mina,' she said. 'Mrs André said you're to go to her room when you arrive. I'm be bringing tea for both of you.'

'Whatever's the matter?' said Auntie when she saw me. 'I knew it wouldn't be any good your going out today. You look terrible.'

I started to tell her about it. She could see I was in a bad way and told me to come and sit next to her on the bed. As I tried to explain I burst into tears again.

She picked up the phone and rang Douglas at once. She wanted to know what he was up to. 'She's breaking her heart here,' she said. 'I want to see you about it.'

He came the next day and saw Auntie alone. She told me later that he had said he could not marry an invalid. He thought I was not strong enough to get married. She gave him short shrift, of course. And in the days and weeks that followed she sustained me in my grief. 'Let it all out, Mina,' she said. 'Just cry it out.'

Then she told me about her life. How sad it was. In particular she told me about one event from her married life when she was about twenty-two. Paul André, her husband, was extremely wealthy. He had interests in several large business concerns, including Austin Cowley and the Goodyear Tyre factory. I only saw him briefly once or twice. He was older than Dagmar and looked every inch the prosperous business man. She had married young and was already estranged from her husband when she became a Christian, but she was still officially living with him. He was not a Christian and she used to spend one day a week in fasting and prayer for him. Then the butler told him that his wife was always reading the Bible and quoting it at him. He said she had religious mania. Mr André used this as a pretext for putting her into a mental hospital.

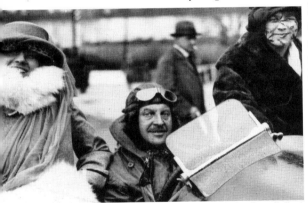

Paul André, associate of Sir Malcolm Campbell

He had influential contacts and knew someone who would undertake the necessary procedures. It was only because the governor of the hospital had his suspicions and acted upon them that she escaped. The governor invited her to take dinner with him. During the course of it he became convinced that she was perfectly sane and saw to it that she was discharged at once.

Shortly after this Mr André arranged a formal separation from his wife, though she managed to strike a hard bargain. He had to provide generous support for her. This included a new car every year, a large allowance and the house on Finchley Road, in addition to money she got out of him for her mission work. Every Wednesday she would be dressed in exquisite chiffon dresses and have a lovely tea waiting for her husband. Wednesday was the day he used to call. I would sometimes wait with her until he came and then discreetly disappear, rejoining her as soon as he had left the house. Quite often, as I came back into her room, her eyes would light up with glee as she showed me a cheque her husband had just written out. 'Look, dear,' she would say, 'I've got another two thousand pounds for my mission.' But she would also spend those Wednesdays in fasting and prayer. Now I knew why.

As she told me of her difficulties with her husband it made me cry all the more. 'Don't worry, dear,' she said to me. 'The Lord wants you for His own. He's got something far better for you.' But it affected me deeply for a long time. I thought I would never be close to any man ever again. In the following months, and even years, my unhappiness and confusion would resurface. Many people had told me I was attractive. Douglas Johnson had always gone on about it. So if I suddenly caught a reflection of myself in the window while riding on a bus, or in a mirror, I would think, 'What's the matter with me?' For a time I became quite embittered and depressed.

I did not go back to work at the mission. Because of my various ailments, which Douglas Johnson had made his excuse for dropping me, I had not been working there for some months. After all that had happened I could not go back now. I stayed at Finchley Road with Auntie.

Some weeks later an invitation to the wedding arrived. I did not want to go.

'Don't be silly,' Auntie said. 'I'll get you a nice frock. You go and show him you don't care. Don't let him see that you're upset.'

She was as good as her word. She bought me a gorgeous, very fashionable, ankle length dress and a big black hat. It really looked nice. She sent me on my way with the words, 'Don't let it worry you. You're well rid of him.' And she said again, 'Remember the Lord has something far better for you.'

So I went. The reception was held in the Portman Rooms in Edgware Road. Douglas Johnson introduced me to his bride. She was called Dorothy. She was a small person. I couldn't think why he was marrying her. But I did as Auntie advised. I tried to appear quite unperturbed by it all, and I think I succeeded.

Many years later – as recently as 1989 – I was staying near Cambridge, on holiday with my husband and a friend. One day we went into Cambridge to shop and came across the Round Church. We went inside to have a look round.

'This is where my heart was broken,' I said to them.

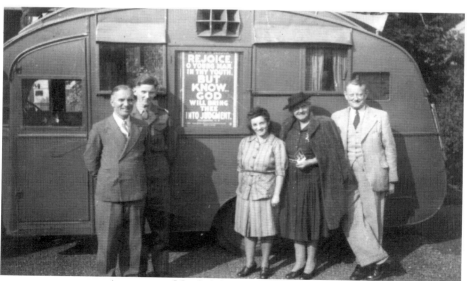

Mrs Andrés mission wagon

5

Mission Denied

Many are called, but few are chosen
Matthew 22.14

Life had to go on – despite Douglas Johnson – and I soon had an opportunity which was to draw my thoughts away from my unhappy love life. I applied for a year's course in tropical medicine at the London Hospital for Tropical Diseases. To my delight, I was accepted and began straightaway.

What a blessing that was. Yet it stirred me up more and more to be a missionary in China. But I was learning that the Lord has His ways: 'O the depth of the riches and wisdom and knowledge of God! How unsearchable are his judgements and how inscrutable are his ways.' (Romans 11.33) His ways, it seemed, were not my ways. His ways were much greater, and He knows the end from the beginning.

I was still living at Mrs André's house. When I was on night duty I would go home – that is, home to Mrs André's – and spend the day there sleeping, curled up on one of the three large couches that she had in her living room. She was becoming more and more like a mother to me, the mother I never had.

We had all sorts of patients at the hospital: natives of the Indian sub-continent, army people, people who had been abroad and had caught malaria or other tropical diseases. One of the patients was a doctor who ran a medical mission in Portugal. His name was Dr Body. Just before he was about to be discharged, he said to me, 'What are you going to do with your life, Miss Staerck? Why are you training?'

'I'm going to be a missionary,' I said.

'Are you? Where?'

'Well, I don't know yet. But I've trained with the China Inland Mission.'

'You know, we're needing a nurse in my Lisbon mission. It's a medical mission and we're worked off our feet.' As he described it I realised it was something like Lansdowne Place, only in Portugal. 'Would you know anybody who might care to come out and work for us?' he asked.

'Yes,' I said. 'I would. As well as my training at the CIM, I'm a qualified nurse and midwife. I think I'd like to help you.'

'That would be marvellous,' he said. 'Look, my wife and I will be staying at Chislehurst for the next few weeks. I've a son at boarding school but he'll be with his friend whose father is a doctor. He loves spending the holidays there. You come out to Chislehurst on your day off. When is it?'

'Thursday.'

'Right. You come out and spend the day with my wife and me on Thursday and we'll be able to tell you all about the mission. Show you pictures too. Then you can have dinner with us in the evening and I'll see that you're back at the station in time for the last train home.'

Thursday came, and the weather was glorious. I set out for Chislehurst by coach – it was a little cheaper than the train. It was a pleasant drive and when I got there I soon found the place where they were staying, a lovely old house.

They gave me such a welcome. They had been talking about it all week, they said, and had been praising the Lord that they would have a nurse to take back with them. They showed me pictures galore and told me all about the work, everything they could think of. The more they spoke about it, the more I was attracted to the idea of working for them.

Then in the evening, over dinner, Dr Body became rather uneasy. Eventually, after exchanging a glance with his wife, he said, 'Now, Mina, I've got something to tell you.'

'Oh, have you?' I said. I couldn't think what he might be going to say.

'Yes. My wife and I went to pick up our son from Harley Street and we of course had a chat with his friend's father. You remember, he's a rather eminent doctor? He asked after our mission. So I told him that our prayers might have been answered, that we had found a nurse and midwife who was interested in our work and who had already been trained for the mission field at the CIM. He asked the name and when I told him, he said, "Oh, I know her. She's a patient of mine."'

'Who's the doctor?' I asked numbly.

'Chave-Cox. You do know him, don't you?'

'Yes, I'm afraid I do,' I replied. My heart was sinking.

'Then you'll probably know what I'm going to tell you. He said to me immediately, "You can't take her." I said, "Why not? She's fully trained and she seems an exceptionally nice girl. I've had nursing from her myself while I was at the Hospital for Tropical Diseases." "Yes, but you can't take her to Lisbon," he said. "She's ill. She'd not last six months." "That's a great pity," I said, "because I was going to ask you to check her health for me." "Well, I'll do that, but I really don't advise that she should go."'

I didn't quite know what to say. This was a bolt from the blue. 'No,' I replied rather lamely. 'He does believe I'm something of an invalid. I can see he might think it rather unwise.'

'My wife and I would be so disappointed,' Dr Body said, 'We'd looked forward so much to your coming to join us.'

I told them then about being turned down for the China Inland Mission. 'But if I've learned nothing else I've learned one thing,' I said. 'Faith in the Lord supplies our every need. So He must have something He wishes for me to do.'

'Yes,' agreed Dr Body. 'He's got some special work for you. He knows what is best for His children. Still, go and see Chave-Cox, won't you? Just in case he changes his mind.'

Privately, I thought there was little chance of that. But we prayed together, and then I said goodbye to Mrs Body, and the doctor saw me back to the coach. The return journey was a sad one. It seemed the Lord did not want me to work as a missionary after all. Yet the call had felt so real.

The outcome of my examination by Dr Chave-Cox was just as I feared it might be. He really rubbed it in. 'You mustn't even think of going to a foreign country,' he said. 'You're not well enough. You're extremely anaemic and you have a heart murmur. Really, you know, you shouldn't be working at all.'

'I've got to work,' I protested vehemently. 'I've got to keep myself.'

But it was no good. The doctor was adamant. Another door to the mission field had just slammed in my face.

While I was at the Hospital for Tropical Diseases I joined a London choir. It was run by a Welshman called Amman Jones. We used to sing in various locations in and around London. Mr Jones took students for personal training at the Wigmore Hall in Central London. One day he suggested that I had my voice trained. I wondered if it would be worthwhile, but he persuaded me it would.

'A trained voice would be no end of good to you, especially as a missionary. I'll give you elocution lessons too. It would help your speaking voice no end.'

So I arranged to have private lessons with him. The idea was that every Tuesday evening I would spend an hour with him in one of the little studios on the first floor of the Wigmore Hall. Because of my busy schedule it was sometimes difficult to get away on time for the lessons, and one Tuesday evening I just could not get away at all. When I turned up the following week he was clearly angry.

'Where were you last Tuesday?' he demanded.

'I just couldn't get off.'

'Mina, give up this nursing lark. Concentrate on singing. You'd do well.'

I didn't believe I had much of a voice, but he had given me good training over the months I had been with him, and I was aware of some improvement – especially in my breathing and the strength of my voice. Another day, not long after, I reached top C. Amman Jones became very excited. He actually jumped up on his chair. 'There! I told you. You should go in for singing, not nursing.'

A few weeks later I lost a tooth. He got upset about that. 'You'll be whistling,' he said. 'A gap in your teeth is no good for singing!'

'Well, I can't help it if a tooth comes out.'

'You'll have to do something about it,' he said.

So I went to the dentist, and had the missing tooth replaced by one on a plate. That appeased him somewhat. But however hard a time he gave me, I knew he had my best interests at heart. I thoroughly enjoyed singing in the choir: it was such a good antidote to the gruelling work at the hospital; and I met several new friends there, one of whom was called Dorothy Thomson. In her late thirties, she was a good ten years older than me, but we got on well and seemed to have a lot in common.

When I was close to finishing my year at the Hospital for Tropical Diseases, I felt I should apply again for some kind of mission work. Perhaps the Lord wished me to do His work not in China but in some other country. So I applied to go to Africa with the Bible Church Mission Society, and went to be interviewed.

I heard nothing from the BCMS, so I applied to a hospital in Walthamstow which was running a six month's course in surgery and emergency operations. I was immediately offered a place, and had accepted it, when news came through that I had also been accepted for the Bible Church Mission Society. With great regret I had to put off taking up the missionary work, hoping I should indeed be able to go off to Africa after I had completed the surgical course.

I started as a night sister at Walthamstow. The experience was extremely helpful. I worked on the surgical wards and the work included a considerable amount of administration: the matron often delegated some of the more arduous paperwork to me. She would also ask me to do her rounds for her.

I was still able to keep up my singing with the choir. Dorothy Thomson and I were becoming good friends. Occasionally she used to invite me home to the double-fronted Georgian house in South Norwood where she lived with her mother. Her father was no longer alive.

Mrs Thomson was a huge woman. She had some connection with the fur trade and she was rather wealthy. They had an elderly maid called Flo. Mrs Thomson treated her like a drudge. Poor Flo had to carry buckets of coal upstairs for the bedroom fires and prepare all their meals. As I got to know Mrs Thomson a little better, I realised she was a real bully.

As a special treat, Dorothy and I would meet regularly for tea at Fortnum and Mason's in Piccadilly before going on to our choir practice. One day she told me that she had received a proposal of marriage from a young man who was the curate at her church. He was called Eric George Wells and he was no older than me – about twenty-seven.

Mrs Thomson was keen on the idea. Dorothy had led an extremely sheltered life, and she was rather timid. She didn't even have a clear idea of where babies came from. I suppose her mother felt that this offer of marriage was too good an opportunity to miss, if Dorothy was to avoid being 'left on the shelf'. Anyway, Dorothy decided to accept the young curate's proposal, and it was agreed that after the wedding they would live at her mother's house.

'Until a baby comes along,' said Dorothy.

'Well, if you do get pregnant,' I said, 'let me know, and if I'm still in the country, I'll come and look after it.'

* * *

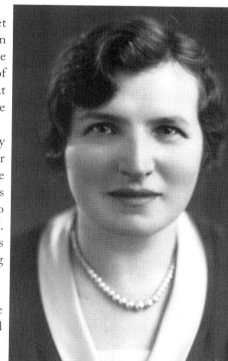

Dorothy Thomson

I was so happy. The BCMS had agreed that I could take up my posting when the six-month placement at Walthamstow was finished. Now the course was nearing its end. All my trunks were packed and ready to leave – everything I needed for life as a nurse on the mission field.

It was a week before I was to set off for Africa. The choir were giving a valedictory concert in my honour to celebrate my becoming a missionary.

The evening before the concert I was on night duty and had to work right through. I was tired but excited at what the next few months might bring. As I came off duty, I happened to bump into the home sister.

'Nurse, what's the matter with you?' she asked.

'Nothing.'

'Yes, there is,' she persisted. 'You look ill.'

'I've just come off night duty. I'm tired, that's all.'

'Come into my office,' she said.

She took my temperature. It was one hundred and three.

'There now,' she said. 'To bed with you. I'm going to ward you.'

'I can't go to bed,' I protested. 'I've got an important engagement this evening.'

'Where?'

'Wigmore Street.'

'You'll have to miss it. You're not going out with a temperature of a hundred and three. You must stay put in bed.'

'Well, I must let them know.'

'I'll see to that,' said the sister.

So I was warded. The year was 1936. My fever was at its height just at the time King George V was dying. Above my bed in the side ward was a radio and I could hear the solemn commentary:

…and now the King's life is slowly drawing to a close…

I hope my life isn't drawing to a close, I thought gloomily.

It turned out that I had pneumonia, and I was really quite poorly. As well as getting that message to the choir, I also had to make sure that the office at the BCMS was informed of my condition. Of course, it meant that I could not take up my post as a missionary. Once again, it seemed, the Lord had shut the door. 'It's quite plain,' I remember thinking, 'He does not want me as a missionary.' I was so upset, and extremely depressed. My faith in the Lord was sorely tried. But I think the feelings were made worse with the delirium of the fever.

Once I was somewhat recovered, Auntie André took me to Bournemouth to recuperate. She said to me, 'The Lord wants you for Himself, dear. He evidently doesn't want you to go abroad, and He has His reasons for it.'

I realised I had to accept it and get on with life.

It was some months before I was fully well again. I don't think I quite realised how poorly I was. I tried filling in my time somehow. I went back to hospital work, and I did another stint at Barnardo's, but at heart I was still confused and upset. The call to the mission field had seemed so real. Did the Lord truly not want me to do His work?

The CIM had a home where retired missionaries and those on furlough could stay. Working at the mission, I had got to know some of the elderly missionaries. One of them came to visit me at Auntie's while I was still recuperating.

She told me of a girl, one of the candidates at my old college, who had been called to the mission field and was now about to leave. But she could not afford to equip herself with the clothing and provisions she would need in China. And there was I, I thought sadly, my trunks still packed with the necessities for life on the field, and my nursing case with all its medical implements and dressings, but with no mission field open to me. On impulse I said, 'Let her have all my things. They're no use to me now.'

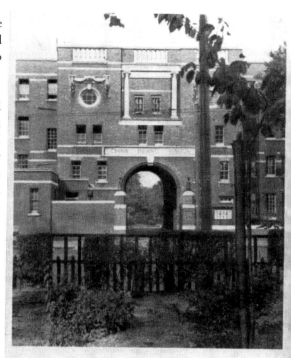

Entrance to the China Inland Mission Newington Green, London, N16

So she took my trunk and my nursing case just as they were. And I thought, maybe this is what the Lord wanted: though I could not go, I am enabling another girl to go.

But the Lord works in mysterious ways. It was not long before another call came for me. A call I could really answer. A call to Malta.

I realised then how the Lord had been preparing me for this work, and I thought of Miss Phillips' words when she had said, 'Get as much experience as you can. Especially in administration.' The Lord had allowed me to do just that. He had barred my way to the mission field, but He had opened other doors. For two years I was to work in Malta. All the experience I had gained was put to the severest test as war raged around us and the island was besieged.

But there were one or two surprises yet in store for me in this country before I was to venture abroad.

6

The Young Parson

Behold, we call those happy who were steadfast
James 5.11

Dorothy Thomson had been married for several months and was now Dorothy Wells. I had spent one or two weekends with them both at their new home. Her young curate had been appointed parson in the Free Church of England with a parish at Wilsborough near Ashford. He seemed a nice fellow.

She must have learned a thing or two in those few months because one day in the spring of 1936, over one of our teas in Fortnum and Mason's, she told me she was pregnant. Home births were common then, and taking me up on my earlier offer, she asked if I would come and live in with them as a private midwife and deliver the baby for her. She also wanted me to be godmother to the child. I told her I would be delighted. I made a note of when the baby was due – late October – and told her I would stay with them for the eight weeks around that date. As the time approached I packed my bags and went to stay.

Her dreadful mother now lived with them at the large Wilsborough manse. She occupied the ground floor of the house. Her poor maid Flo had come too and had a room at the back near the kitchen and scullery. Dorothy and Eric had the upstairs to themselves. Their bedroom was at the top of the stairs.

Because her mother had been so protective of her and had never let her soil her hands with washing up or cleaning the house, Dorothy had no idea of running a home. I more or less had to teach her the rudiments of keeping house. That wasn't all I had to teach her. She had no idea what was involved in giving birth. She had an idea the baby would somehow appear through her belly-button. I had to school her in the various aspects of what she should expect. As the day drew near she grew increasingly nervous but was comforted to know I would be on hand when the time came.

It was a long, painful labour. Eric of course was terribly anxious. He didn't come into the bedroom, but it must have been worse for him hearing Dorothy's cries and being able to do nothing about it. I kept him occupied running up and down the stairs, helping Flo fetch the hot water, towels and extra linen. As usual, Mrs Thomson was more hindrance than help. When I asked Eric to ring for the doctor, she came up and plonked herself on the edge of Dorothy's bed. She was a huge woman, and the fur coat she invariably wore made her look bigger still.

'Oh, Mrs Thomson,' I said, 'don't sit there. Will you sit on a chair?'

'I'm going to sit here and see my daughter through.'

'You'll hinder doctor when he comes. He won't be able to do his work properly. And you'll hinder me in looking after Dorothy. Please sit on a chair.'

But she would not budge. She was a difficult person, brusque and offensive when not getting her own way. This really would not do, I thought, but I did have a scheme in mind to get her out of the way. The next time Eric came up with water, I went out and spoke to him quietly on the landing.

'Eric, we must get Mrs Thomson back downstairs. Ask Flo to say she's wanted, say anything you like, as long as we get her out of this room. Otherwise I cannot be responsible for what might happen.'

Alarmed, he went back downstairs, and a few moments later Flo was at the door. 'Madam, you're wanted on the phone.'

'Don't bother me now, Flo,' said Mrs Thomson. 'You see to it. Tell them my daughter's in labour.'

But Flo persisted, and Mrs Thomson was persuaded to take the imaginary call in her study. As soon as she had picked up the phone, Eric pulled the door to and locked her in. When she realised the deceit she was furious. She banged on the door and shouted, but we kept her shut in down there while the doctor arrived and he and I attended to Dorothy.

Doctor Milne was a friend of Eric's. He found that Dorothy had fibroids and they were obstructing the birth canal. Together, we saw Dorothy through. Afterwards he told Eric that he owed the life of his wife and son to me. I don't know how true that was, but Eric and Dorothy were certainly grateful to me for attending at the birth. They even asked me to choose a name for the child. I suggested John, and so that was what the little boy was called. John Wells.

Mrs Thomson was less grateful. She never forgave me the trick I'd played on her. Nor, I think, did she forgive Eric. Nevertheless, her daughter was safe and the proud mother of a healthy son. For the next few weeks I stayed with the family as agreed, to ensure that both mother and son made good progress.

One morning I was having breakfast in Dorothy's bedroom. She was in bed and Eric was sitting with us having coffee. As usual, Flo came up with tea and toast and the morning post. There was a letter for me, redirected from Auntie's. It was from Douglas Johnson of all people. It began with one of his pet names for me:

Dear Puss, Dorothy has gone up to bed and I can't get you out of my mind. So I thought I'd write to you. The grass is up to the window sills. I ought to be cutting it, but I can't be bothered. All I can think of is you...

At the bottom he had written,

Now burn this letter!

It brought back the whole situation. I thought I had left it all behind me but the memories came flooding back. Tears sprang into my eyes. I could not conceal them.

'What's the matter?' Eric asked.

I tried to explain a little of what had happened and showed them the letter. Eric grew angry for me.

'There's only one thing to be done with this,' he said, and he tore it into little pieces and threw it in the fire. He turned to me and took my hand.

'Now, Mina, listen to me. You're not to let this experience spoil your life. Don't turn away from other men. I know the Lord will have somebody for you.'

'I just cannot understand the man,' I said. 'How could he write to me like this when he's married. His poor wife.' Dorothy looked on wide-eyed in disbelief at such behaviour and nodded in agreement.

'He's not worth you, Mina,' said Eric. 'He's not worth your even thinking about him.'

In the weeks and months that followed, even after I had left them, Eric continued to be concerned I should meet the right man. As I was to be a godmother I returned to their house for John's christening. They had chosen some other friends of theirs, a minister and his wife, to be one set of godparents. The other godfather was an old friend of Eric's, a Frenchman.

'I'm going to get you off with this friend of mine,' said Eric, before they had all arrived. 'You'll see. You'll be the perfect wife for him.'

'Oh, you mustn't worry about me,' I replied.

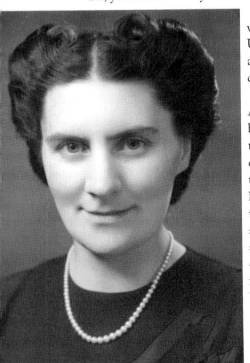

I must admit I was a little intrigued as to what this Frenchman would be like. Unfortunately, he made no impression on me at all. They talked French all the time and I couldn't understand a word.

After my stay with Dorothy and Eric, I went back to living with Auntie Dagmar. She was treating me more and more like her own daughter. She would often come back from her travels with an outfit for me to try on. She'd happened to see it in a shop window, she would tell me, and found an assistant of about my size and got her to try it on. If Auntie liked what she saw, she would buy it for me. On one occasion she came back with a maroon coat with matching beaver collar and hat. It fitted beautifully, and suited me I think.

I suppose I must have cut rather a stylish figure at that time. Auntie made sure I was dressed well all the time I was with her, in outfits I would never have been able to afford. All her money came from her husband, of course. Whenever Christmas was approaching she would tell him she wanted such and such an amount. 'For my mothers,' she said. This was what she called her mission people.

She was a strong-willed woman. She was also impulsive. On her birthday – the eleventh of November, Remembrance Day – there was a spanking new car outside her door which her husband had exchanged for the previous one. She liked cars, especially big cars. 'We're spending a couple of days at the cottage,' she said, 'just you and me,' and we set off for Sutton in the new car.

At the back of her cottage in Sutton there was a big garden. Part of it was choked with lilies. It was a tangled untidy mess. We had often wondered how we could make it neater. Auntie now had an idea. 'We're going to dig it all up and put concrete over it. Then we can have a table and chairs out here.'

So the day after we arrived we set about pulling up all the lilies. It took a whole morning. She then went off in her car and came back with a sackful of cement and a sackful of sand and gravel. 'Now,' she said, 'It's got to be three of one and one of the other. That's what the man at the shop said.'

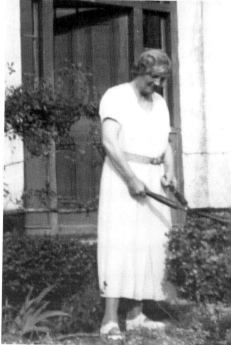

We shovelled the sand and gravel and cement together, kept adding water, and slopped it all about with a spade. We were making a terrible mess, but Auntie always went at everything with a great will and we were thoroughly enjoying ourselves. She never did anything without getting smudges on her face, and I was the same. The white cement got everywhere. Suddenly, we heard a car draw up at the front of the cottage. It was her husband.

'Keep down,' she whispered.

Mr André strode through the gate and round to the rear entrance without seeing us.

'I'd better go and see him, I suppose,' she said, wiping her cement-encrusted hands on the old tunic she had on. 'Pray, dear.'

He was furious when he saw what we had

Auntie in her cottage garden

been doing. 'Don't I allow you enough that you've got to do this sort of thing yourself? Why didn't you get some proper workers to do it?'

I dreamed, that night, of pulling up lilies. But we finished the job. After a few days the concrete was dry. Auntie found a table and chairs and set them out, and placed a big parasol over them so we could sit in the shade and enjoy the garden from what had once been the tangles of an old patch of lilies.

With the New Year I felt it was time to start looking for another job. Auntie was almost too good to me: I felt the need to be independent, to support myself and extend my experience of nursing. Despite Chave-Cox's dire warnings about the state of my health, I felt I must stand on my own two feet and start earning my own living again. There was an advert in *Nursing Mirror* for a holiday relief sister at the Kent and Sussex Hospital, Tunbridge Wells. I applied and was accepted.

The hospital had been built only a few years earlier and was bang up to date. Since I was filling in for sisters on each of the wards in succession as they took their breaks, it meant that I gained a thorough experience of a variety of medical, surgical and nursing procedures.

I so enjoyed the work. The hospital had been well designed and I liked the modern arrangement of the wards within the building. When I arrived, the Gynaecology ward was being upgraded. It consisted of twenty beds and one private room. At one end was the Outpatients department with its examinations room and small clinic where emergency treatment could be administered. At the further end was a full operating theatre for more major surgery, such as caesarean section. I took over as relief on Gynaecology just as this new work was being completed. After a week or two the matron called me to her office.

'How do you enjoy working on the new ward, Sister Staerck?' she asked.

'Very much,' I told her.

'Well, I want to offer you the position of full-time sister there. If you'd like to take it, it's yours.'

'Oh yes, I would.' My reply was immediate. I knew how useful such experience would be for the mission field – for that was still my long term aim.

So I became the sister on the new gynaecological ward. I was able to employ my midwifery to the full, and I loved every baby I delivered. I had good staff, and the doctors were co-operative – which is not always the case, I have found!

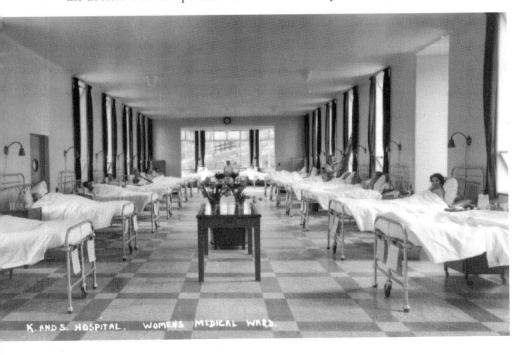

K. AND S. HOSPITAL. WOMENS MEDICAL WARD.

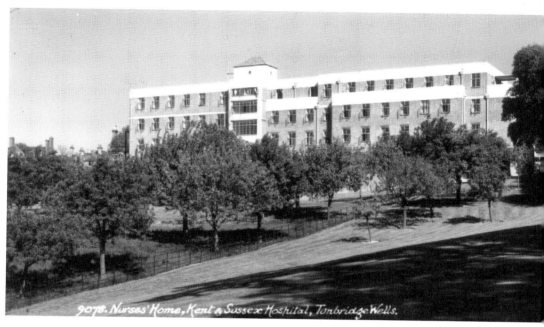

9078. Nurses' Home, Kent & Sussex Hospital, Tunbridge Wells.

The nurses' accommodation was new and comfortable, with fine views of the surrounding countryside, and I had soon made many friends. At the end of the day we often met in each others' rooms to chat. I became particularly friendly with the ward sister of the medical department. Funnily enough, her surname was Ward. Her first name was Anne. She was a Roman Catholic. Whenever she was off duty she would go to her church to pray. For hours on end we would discuss our different religions. Anne would talk about Catholicism and try to win me over to it, and I spoke of my spiritual understanding and tried to explain how my faith in the Lord had arisen. It was a case of RC versus Free Church.

One day she said to me, 'You know, I'll be going away soon.'

I asked her where she was going.

'I'm a novice of the Carmelite order. One day soon I'll be leaving here to take up my calling. I can't tell you where I'm going, and I won't be able to write to let you know anything about it. It's a silent order. We are not allowed to communicate with anyone once we are there.'

'That's a great pity,' I said. 'You're such a good sister. Don't you think it's a waste of your hospital experience?'

'No. It won't be a waste. Wherever I'm sent I shall always continue my nursing. I shall be doing it as a member of the Carmelite order, that's all. That's the only difference. But it's an important one.'

We had one patient who had a difficult delivery of her baby. She nearly lost her life, and we all had to work hard. Finally she had a caesarean. Mercifully, both she and the baby survived the operation. It was my weekend off, so when the emergency was over I prepared to leave, telling the staff nurse to keep an eye on the mother.

When I returned on Sunday evening I called in at the ward. Things seemed quiet enough, and I went off to unpack in my room. As I got there the staff nurse arrived. 'Oh, sister, I've sad news. Our caesarean patient had a relapse – a pulmonary embolism. We lost her.'

This was such a shock to me. I had left for my weekend leave thinking the woman completely out of danger. The nurse went to resume her duties, then popped her head back round the door. 'Did you manage to catch Sister Ward?'

'No,' I said.

'She was asking for you before she went. She's left us, you know.'

Then I saw that on my table there was a big pot of white tulips. Tucked inside was a card with just one word written on it: 'Goodbye'. My friend had gone.

The shock at the loss of my patient deepened now into a greater sorrow as this further loss sunk in. Not only had I lost a friend – for she was as good as lost to me in the silence of the Carmelites – but she was also lost to the hospital, and she had been such a good sister, running her ward so well. Again I felt what a waste it was – that lovely person going where she was not allowed to talk or write or visit her former friends and colleagues, or even receive letters or visits from us. She was just gone, and I had no idea where.

I stayed at the Kent and Sussex for more than a year. Auntie would come up to see me from time to time. My off-duty days were usually Thursday and Friday, and often I would spend them with her in her new house in Rosalind Road, Richmond.

To get to Richmond from Tunbridge Wells, I had to go to Charing Cross and change. One mid-morning, I was just walking along the platform at Charing Cross to catch the Richmond train when who should be there but Dorothy's young curate, the Reverend Eric Wells. 'Good gracious!' I said.

'Yes, this is a marvellous accident,' he said, 'What are you doing here? Come and have a tea with me.'

'I'm sorry. I can't, Eric. Auntie's expecting me in Richmond. I'm having a meal there.'

'Aw, come along,' he said, 'There's a nice little restaurant I know round the corner on Charing Cross Road. Come and have a bite to eat.'

I found him difficult to refuse – it was so good to see him again. He brought me to what looked like a hotel. On the first floor was a high-class restaurant. He ordered lunch for us both and asked for a bottle of claret. It was the first time I had drunk wine.

He told me all about Dorothy and the baby, how they were getting on, and we giggled when we remembered how we had locked Mrs Thomson in her room. We passed a most enjoyable couple of hours, eating the splendid meal and chatting about this and that. Then I suddenly remembered the time and realised I had better catch my train to Richmond.

'Give my love to Dorothy, won't you?' I called as I ran for the train.

'I certainly will,' he shouted after me.

Every Thursday after that we would invariably bump into each other. One day, since it was so fine, he suggested we go for a bus ride.

'Let's go to Sevenoaks,' he said. 'It's beautiful there. Do you know it?'

So we caught a bus and when we got there we found that the Forestry Commission had been busy. Many of the oaks were being cut down. It was very pleasant countryside and we walked for a time through the wood until we came to a clearing. A big oak tree was lying on its side.

'Let's sit here,' Eric suggested.

The sun came dappled through leaves and branches and we chatted pleasantly for a while. I was asking about Dorothy and how she and the baby were, when suddenly he leaned forward and kissed me.

'Oh, Mina, you know I love you.'

I was shocked.

'You mustn't,' I said. 'You can't love me. You're already married. I'd never come between any man and his wife.'

'Oh, don't be like that,' he said. 'I think we were made for each other.'

'Well, I don't. You've got a lovely wife and a lovely baby.'

'Oh, but Mina, I took to you the first moment I saw you. Surely you know that.'

'No, I don't know that. I've never even thought of it.'

This was true, though I must have been rather naive at the time. But now an incident came back to me that somehow fell into place. While I was staying with them at Wilsborough, I had come across an envelope propped up on the mantelpiece, along with a pair of scissors. It was addressed to me. Inside had been a note: 'Cut a lock of your hair and put it in here. Eric.'

I was so busy at the time that I didn't think all that much about it. I had done as he requested. I didn't know what else to do. But I mentioned nothing about it to anyone, not to him, nor to Dorothy. Nothing further had been said, and I had soon forgotten all about it. Eric, evidently, had not.

'I've loved you since the first time I met you,' Eric was saying. 'I can't help it. I want to shout it from the treetops.'

He stood up, and flung his arms out wide. 'I LOVE YOU!' he shouted.

I was appalled. 'No! You mustn't love me,' I said to him firmly. 'I'm not coming between you and Dorothy. You've got a little son to think of now. You mustn't even think of loving me!'

He looked at me then for a long while and finally realised that I really meant it.

'When I'm free,' he said, 'I shall search to the ends of the earth to find you.'

We returned to Charing Cross Road in embarrassed silence. I caught my Richmond train thinking I must never see him again.

After that day we no longer bumped into to each other at the station. A little time later I heard that Dorothy, Eric and their little son John had moved from Ashford to a vicarage attached to a church in Teddington. The young parson had taken up a new post.

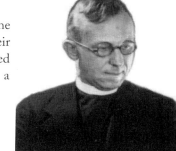

The Reverend Eric Wells

7

Malta

He trains my hands for war…
Psalm 18.34

There were rumblings and rumours of war. Hitler was in the ascendant. I joined the Queen Alexander Naval Nursing Service (Territorials). In the event of war I could be called up to serve as a nurse. Reluctant though I was to leave the Kent and Sussex where I had been so happy, I felt I must be ready to face up to the changes war might bring.

The day came when I received a letter from the Ministry of Defence. It instructed all Territorials to prepare to resign their hospital posts since the Ministry would soon be requiring their services. Within a matter of weeks I was informed that the Merchant Service Christian Friends Society needed an assistant matron at the King George V Merchant Seamen's Memorial Hospital in Valletta, the capital of Malta. Taking the bit between my teeth, I asked for more information. A letter by return invited me to meet the secretary at the MSCFS's London headquarters on Vauxhall Bridge Road.

While waiting to go in for the interview I met a young gentleman, a doctor who had offered himself for a post at the same hospital. His was the interview before mine. Once he was finished it was my turn to go in and hear all about the work. The post of assistant matron was becoming available because the incumbent – her name was Joyce Barnes – was about to be married. Her prospective husband was the supervisor of the milk pasteurising plant. Being Malta, it was goat's milk of course.

They told me during the interview that they would be glad to have me take over as assistant matron. The young doctor who had preceded me had also been accepted and they felt it would be a good idea, as we would be working together, to make the journey to Malta together. The date they suggested was only a week away – the first of May 1939.

I pointed out that this might be difficult since I had to give a month's notice at the Kent and Sussex. But I promised to have a word with the matron and see if anything could be done.

The next day I arranged to see the matron and explained the situation.

'Oh, my dear,' she said, 'Malta is in a strategic position if the war should escalate. Do you think you are wise taking up this post?'

'I know it might be difficult, but for me it will be a kind of missionary work. I really do feel I must take up the challenge. The trouble is the month's notice.'

She smiled at me kindly.

'Well, you've got two weeks' vacation owing to you, and I know you put in a lot of additional hours when Gynaecology was being upgraded. Leave it with me. I'll speak to the committee. Let's see what they say.'

The next morning she sent for me. 'I've seen the committee,' she said, 'and the chairman thinks we should let you have the extra time.'

Immediately I rang through to the Christian Friends Society and confirmed that I should be free to take up my post in Malta on the date they had in mind. That night I went home happy, convinced that the Lord was leading me.

After finishing at the Kent and Sussex, I moved back in with Auntie. She was now living in a luxurious new service flat near the Dorchester Hotel in Park Lane.

I had to let all my friends know of my imminent departure, and I could not, of course, exclude Eric and Dorothy Wells. Eric expressed great sadness that I should be leaving the country on such a potentially dangerous mission. Given the situation between us, however, it seemed right that I should get as far away from him as possible. I was fond of him, but I was fond of Dorothy as well. It was the fairest thing for her, did she but know it.

The morning I was to leave, the postman brought me a package. I opened it in front of Auntie. It contained a contact sheet of photos and a gold signet ring. There was also a note:

You're breaking my heart. But I shall continue to write and to think of you. Eric.

The photos were all of him. I looked at the ring. The inscription appeared to be a series of swirls. Then the pattern fell into place – the letters *E* and *M* intertwined. I slid it over my finger. It fitted perfectly. I decided to keep it.

The idea had been that I should fly to Rome and travel on from there. But because of the uncertainties and complications brought about by Mussolini entering the war on Germany's side, the route had to be changed. Now I had to leave, less glamorously, from Victoria station. I was not now to be travelling with the young doctor: he was making his own way there. So on the first of May at two-thirty in the afternoon I waved goodbye to Auntie Dagmar as the train bound for Rome moved out of the station.

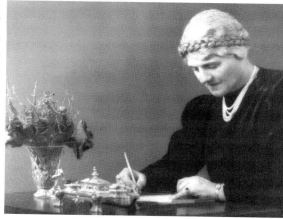

Mrs Dagmar André

The train carriages were made up of small compartments of six or eight seats. Having located my compartment and seat, I quickly discovered that opposite me was a nurse who was also in the Queen Alexander Naval Nursing Service and travelling to Malta. Her name was Barbara Tyndale Biscoe. On that long journey we became well acquainted and eventually became firm friends.

We crossed the Channel and travelled through France. At Paris we were held up in a siding as another train passed us, full of high-spirited Tommies, shouting and singing, making their way to the front. Our train remained in the siding for several hours as an air raid raged to the south of Paris. Eventually the all-clear came and we were able to continue our journey towards Marseilles. When we got there, the station was full of men with blankets and stretchers. News had reached them of the heavy bombardment over Paris. A train – it was thought to be our train – had suffered a direct hit with many casualties. We soon discovered it was the train full of soldiers that had received the direct hit. Mercifully we had been spared, but that night our thoughts were with those poor soldiers. Their fates and ours could so easily have been reversed.

At Marseilles we boarded a ship, the *Stranraer*. We were given a hot meal and blankets to wrap ourselves up in. I was so thankful to the Lord for His care and protection. Just that morning I had read in the Daily Light: 'Though the mountains fall into the sea, yet will I be with you. I will be with you even unto the end of the world.' The truth of that message came home to me. He was going before.

As we arrived at Malta and entered the Grand Harbour of Valletta, we stood on the deck to get the first glimpse of our destination. The sun was shining, bells were ringing, bands were playing. There were crowds of people on the quayside. I said to Barbara, 'Seems as though they're giving us a welcome.'

But as we came nearer we could see many groups of women who appeared to be wailing and sobbing. The bands and the bells and the crowds were not there to welcome us. We learned, as we waited to disembark, that Malta was sending its first battalion of men off to war. One of the troopships had just left the harbour.

Waiting on the quay to meet us was the matron of the King George V Hospital and the young doctor whom I'd met at my interview. He was a Dubliner, and his name was Eric Doyle. I introduced Barbara to them both.

When Eric shook my hand he noticed the signet ring I was wearing.

'What's that?' he enquired.

'Oh, a friend gave it me. He's upset because I'm coming to Malta.'

I discovered only later – after the doctor and I had got to know each other a little better – that Eric Wells had written to Eric Doyle, claiming I was going to Malta to get away from him. He had written:

> …I love her, and if anything should happen to her I could never forgive myself. So I want you to look after her for me…

Barbara was to be working at Bighi, Malta's naval hospital. It was on the other side of the Grand Harbour from the King George V Hospital and a small cruiser had been laid on to take her across. As we parted she said, 'We're working so near each other, we must meet up. Let's keep in touch.'

On the way to our hospital Eric said, 'It's going to be a tough job, you know.'

'I know,' I replied. 'But I've had a comforting message from the Lord. He is going before.'

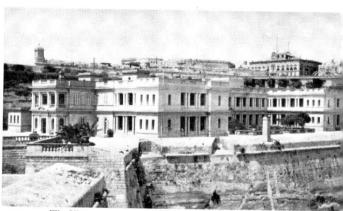

The King George V Merchant Seamen's Memorial Hospital, Malta

The hospital – which everyone referred to as the KG5 – was in an outlying district called Floriana. It was a pleasant white building, containing around a hundred beds and dating from the First World War, when it had been bombed and rebuilt. It was in memory of this that it had received King George V's name.

Eric was a keen Christian. 'I'm glad you've come,' he said, when I had unpacked and settled in. 'I've been looking forward to working with you.'

We took to each other at once and I found him a great support in the difficult weeks and months ahead.

My room was on the first floor, with a breathtaking view of the Grand Harbour. There were very few ships in the harbour. Normally, I was told, the port would be full of merchant vessels coming and going, discharging their cargo and loading up again. The war had put a stop to that. From my balcony I could see the young sailors unable to set sail. They spent the time lazing by the harbour, sunning their already bronzed bodies on the quayside, or diving from the harbour wall and swimming in the calm blue waters.

I could also look down on the hospital's sunken garden. I came to love that garden. All sorts of beautiful flowers blossomed there. I especially remember the hibiscus and the mimosa. In the Maltese climate they bloomed four times a year. Then the perfume from the mimosa filled the air. From my window I could look down on the large clusters of pink and purple mimosa flowers. Sitting or walking in the garden I could enjoy the shade of its feathery foliage. But if one so much as touched them, the leaves would fold up and collapse.

Just a few days after I arrived, the matron of the hospital was taken ill. It was discovered she had cancer and required treatment in England. The waters around Malta were becoming increasingly dangerous, but she managed to go with a convoy of ships that was bound for Great Britain and I was promoted to the post of matron in her place.

There was a medical superintendent at the hospital by the name of Captain Curry. He too became poorly and had to retire. Eric Doyle was appointed to this senior post. Within weeks of our arrival, as war clouds darkened on the not-too-distant horizon, the sole responsibility for running the hospital had fallen to Eric and myself.

Because of the threat of bombardment the first thing we did was to draw up a rota, so that each person would have a clearly defined responsibility. Mr Gordon, the pharmacist, started on an inventory of his drugs to see how long supplies might last. I had a trained staff of six nursing sisters – all qualified SRNs; the rest of the nursing staff were voluntary assistants, mainly daughters of the dock workers. Each of the sisters had a ward to look after and it was their job to discover which of the patients could be moved in the event of emergency.

The sisters' accommodation and nurses' lounge was on the first floor, along the corridor from my room. Each of the rooms, like mine, had a balcony. The balcony for the nurses' lounge was large and had on it a cage containing linnets and canaries. We hadn't forgotten these birds in drawing up our contingency plans. When the warning of bombardment came it was the first duty of whichever of the staff was in the lounge to put a black cover over the cage and to wheel it into the relative safety of the lounge. Only then could that member of staff join the rest of us in seeing to the safety of the patients.

Lieutenant-General Sir William Dobbie had only recently been appointed Governor of the Island. He was a good man and concerned that our preparations for war should be effective. Inside the entrance of the hospital was a large marble staircase. The only place that provided some shelter in an air raid was under these stairs. A wall of sandbags was built up to give additional protection. When the general visited us and saw our makeshift shelter he said, 'This is dangerous. Should there be a direct hit on the hospital, the stairs might give way. It could cause serious injury.'

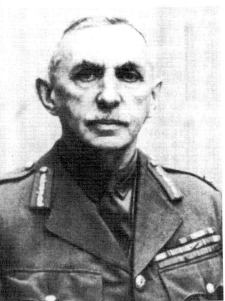

General Sir William Dobbie, Governor of Malta

We pointed out that this was the best shelter available to us.

'You must have a shelter built,' he said. 'I'll see to it.'

Within a day or two workers came along with their tools, and with their own food: a Maltese loaf, a couple of ounces of olive oil poured into a hole in the bread, garnished with garlic and onions. Our chef provided them with a drink to go with it. The chef was Maltese, a little tub of a man, about four-and-a-half foot in height and probably as much round. It was his job in the event of a raid to see that the cooking gas and water supply were switched off as soon as the warning came. So, gradually, we prepared for the onslaught that we knew must come. We held a service every day in each of the wards, to pray for our deliverance. Eric and I took turns to lead it.

When I had arrived there were clear signs of discontent and tension among the sisters. The petty squabbling was beginning to affect morale. I felt now was the time to do something about it. I called the staff together and explained to them the difficulty we were in. We must have a strict routine and follow it closely. It was essential that our rota of responsibilities was adhered to. Above all, I told them, we must be compassionate to each other in these difficult times or it would be the patients who would suffer.

They weren't ready to be convinced at first. 'We've heard all this before,' came the reply. 'Love thy neighbour, etcetera, etcetera.'

'It isn't just a case of loving your neighbour,' I said. 'You're here to do a job. And unless you get on with each other that job will not be carried out properly. It will reflect badly on the patients. You must be of high integrity and sympathetic to each other. Especially to the patients.'

I don't know if they took much of this in, but it was a start.

On Saturday nights we always had a special meal which I encouraged the ward sisters to attend if they could. The chef displayed great enterprise and inventiveness, given the restricted range of food he had to choose from. This was my first time in a foreign country and I found some of his dishes rather exotic. We might start off with minestrone soup served with a bowl of powdered Parmesan cheese to sprinkle over it. He sometimes used to make pigeon pie – pigeons were plentiful, if nothing else was – and in the pie there would also be aubergine, which was a vegetable I had not known before I came to Malta. Aubergine was not widely available in Britain then – at least, I had not come across it. When I first discovered it in the food the chef served up, I imagined he was experimenting with some sort of bitter mushroom he had found in the kitchen gardens.

There were an orange tree and a lemon tree in the kitchen garden. I used to love picking the large and juicy fruit. The Saturday following my talk with the sisters, I took an orange for every person at table, made four incisions in each and turned back the skin to give the impression of petals, revealing the fruit within. I placed one orange at each setting. Then I picked the scarlet hibiscus flowers and arranged them in a black bowl I had found, placing it in the centre of the table. I felt that making an effort like this once a week would raise our spirits and give us something to look forward to. It certainly helped this particular Saturday. The sisters saw that I was trying to brighten things up for them and the atmosphere became less fraught.

On the tenth of June 1939 Italy declared war on the Allies. Malta was in the firing line but psychologically the little island community was not ready for it. They could not bring themselves to believe that Italy would fight against them. There was so much intermarriage between the Maltese and the Italians. Family would be fighting family. It was unthinkable. But that was the way it turned out.

It was not long before we were coming under weekly bombardment, often during the night. Every bomb that fell in the vicinity of the Grand Harbour

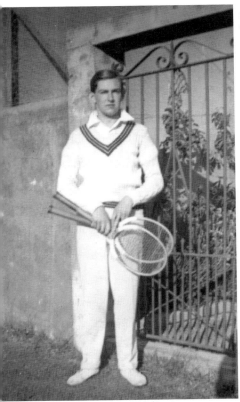

A break for tennis with Dr Eric Doyle

shattered windows in our hospital. Barbara Tyndale Biscoe's hospital, across the other side of the harbour, was the first to receive a direct hit. Taken up with the war preparations, we had not been in touch with her since the day of our arrival. When we heard what had happened, Eric immediately phoned Bighi Hospital to find out how Barbara was.

She was absolutely fine and took the opportunity of inviting us over to Bighi for a game of tennis. She even arranged for a cruiser to pick us up and take us across the harbour. As a big naval hospital, Bighi had a swimming pool as well as tennis courts. We were all in need of an occasional break from routine and Eric and I were soon spending much of our free time there. It made a welcome change from the workload at the hospital which became heavier as the bombing raids became more frequent.

General Dobbie and his men provided much appreciated assistance in standing up to the increasing bombardments. During heavy air raids, the general would personally arrive with his retinue and help us move the beds to the safer areas and into the shelter that the workmen had dug into the sandstone rock under the hospital.

Because there had been little preparation for war among the population at large, few bomb shelters had been built. As a rudimentary measure, the granaries were opened up. It was pitiful to see people rushing to these and climbing down into them whenever the sirens sounded, for they offered little protection.

One naval officer who would come to see us and lend a hand whenever his ship got through was Lieutenant Frederick Plenty. He was on one of the battle cruisers that gave protection to merchant ships carrying much needed food and supplies between Malta and other Allied countries. He and Eric became good friends. We called him Freddy.

He turned up rather ill one day with bronchitis. He had eaten little for several days because his throat was so sore. Eric examined him and took Freddy up to his own room. When he came back down he said to me, 'I've had to put Freddy to bed. He's running a high temperature and he's weak. Can you get him some food?'

I went to the kitchens and took Freddy some soup and some ice cream – food that would slip down his throat without causing too much discomfort. He was so weak I had to spoonfeed him. I was sitting on the edge of the bed doing this, when Eric came in to see how his patient was. Freddy, though he found it difficult to talk, did seem to be responding well.

'For pity's sake, matron, he's not meant to be enjoying it,' joked Eric in his Dublin brogue. 'This is meant to be medical treatment. Stop looking at him like that. It's more than any man can bear.'

KG5 was gradually filling up with the local people, and from time to time merchant seamen and airmen would be brought in. One day a Finnish ship arrived in the harbour. It had been attacked when it was nearing Malta. The entire crew of twenty-two had sustained injury and needed attention. The captain had received wounds to his eyes.

That night we had a terrible air raid. We managed to get all the patients, new and old, into the shelter which had only just been completed. It was the first time we had been down there. The smell of garlic from the workmen's lunches still hung around the place.

It was rather grim. The captain was in urgent need of medical attention. He lay in a corner of the shelter as Eric used a magnet to extract the slivers of metal from his eyes. In another corner was a pregnant Maltese woman in the first stages of labour. The members of our domestic staff became somewhat hysterical as the bombs started to explode overhead. 'It's the end,' they wailed. 'It's the end of the world.' They were telling their rosaries and calling out, 'Ave Maria, save us, save us!' and causing unease among the rest of the patients.

I said to the ward sisters, 'We can't do with all this. Let's join together and sing a chorus.' And so that's what we did and it calmed us all down. We sang:

> Turn your eyes upon Jesus.
> Look full in His wonderful face
> And the things of earth will grow strangely dim
> In the light of His glory and grace.

By the time the baby was born there was no water left to clean it with. But the mother urinated shortly after giving birth, and we were able to make use of this sterile liquid to clean its little face and eyes.

Finally the air raid abated and we got the patients safely back to the wards. We even had one extra – the little baby who was delivered in the night. Taking the service the following day, Eric referred to the goodness of the Lord. We were indeed in His hands, he said, and He would never let us go. He was the Almighty God, the Great One, victorious over all evil.

I was in attendance a few days later when Eric came to treat the captain's eyes again. 'I'm just going to lift your bandage to have a look,' he said, 'but I don't want you to open your eyes. It's too early yet.'

As Eric carried out his examination the captain said, 'You know, when those girls were singing *Turn Your Eyes Upon Jesus*, I did turn my eyes upon Him. So I'm not worried. Even if I lose the sight of my eyes, I shall have spiritual sight.'

Thus, even out of that terrible night, came some good. The captain became a strong Christian and was a great witness of God's loving care. And against all the odds his sight was saved.

There were two or three raids every week, and so it went on through the whole of the following two years. It was a terrible test of endurance and faith. Because the convoys were unable to get through with the usual supplies, people were beginning to starve. There was too little food grown on the island to sustain the whole population. Quite early on I realised how serious things were getting when one day the general rang me and said, 'Matron, I want you to get whatever men you can spare and send them down to the quay. We believe a convoy is getting through. We must be ready to make the most of it. They'll be bringing in supplies, God willing, but we must off-load it all as quickly as possible. Also, can I ask you to send along as many bottles of goat's milk and packs of sandwiches as you have to spare? We're going to take this opportunity of getting some of the women and children off the island. It may be their last chance of survival. We'll need to pack them up with something to sustain them.'

I had the food prepared. Eric – together with the pharmacist, the chef and the gardener – took it down to the quay. The convoy made safely into port, the much needed supplies were unloaded and as the ships put out to sea again many of the island's women and children went with them – on route to safer shores. The same day Lady Dobbie found two large sausages in her pantry. She sent them over to the hospital and with those, and the extra supplies brought back from the convoy, our diet was made a little more interesting for the next few days.

Despite the hardship, some wonderful things happened which served to demonstrate to us the goodness of the Lord. On Malta the heavy rains come late in the year. Terrace upon terrace had been constructed over the centuries to prevent the topsoil being washed away into the sea. That year things were different. The rains began in early September. It started with huge hailstones, as large as ping-pong balls, pelting down on to the still unharvested crops. The people were becoming excited and upset. They were superstitious and, what with the horrors the war had brought, felt it betokened the end.

Some of our domestic staff were on the flat roof when the unnatural hailstones came thundering down. They saw it as a forewarning of the evil to come, and cried out in anguish. Eric and I went up on to the roof to see for ourselves. Large pellets of ice, hard as pebbles, pelted painfully down on us. Looking across the harbour we could see nothing, visibility was so bad. The sky was black. Then, as suddenly as it had started, the storm abated and the darkness lifted.

'Look,' said Eric, pointing out to sea. Over the water had appeared a gigantic rainbow, from one side of the harbour to the other. 'The bow in the clouds. It's a sign that the Lord is with us.'

A cargo ship passed into harbour under the rainbow arch. It had survived the heavy storm and was bringing in much needed food and supplies. The Lord had kept His promise to us as He did to Noah in Genesis 9.11-13: 'And I will establish my covenant with you; neither shall all flesh be cut off any more by the waters…I do set my bow in the cloud and it shall be for a token of a covenant.'

Christmas came and went, and we were soon into a new year – 1942. The onslaught grew more intense. Despite everything, we still managed to make some time for ourselves. Without such breaks, I think it would have been impossible to go on. In early April the weather was glorious and we felt we should take full advantage of our one day off duty.

On the far side of the island there was a town called Boschetto. A building was set aside there as a kind of recreational centre for the use of the hospital staff when they needed a break. Barbara, Eric and I decided to brave the constant air raids and walk across the island to it, picnicking on the way. Barbara packed the frugal sandwiches, and Eric and I went to the market to buy fruit – still in plentiful supply because it grew in such abundance on the island.

The island is nine miles wide and thirteen in length. That day we walked the breadth of Malta, dodging the bombs. Under normal conditions it should have taken us three or four hours, but that day it took us a lot longer. Whenever we heard the bombers coming we looked for the nearest shelter and raced for it. It was dangerous, but somehow, after being cooped up in the hospital for so long, exhilarating too.

The day was fine with the clear blue skies of early spring, warm but not too hot. When at last we were nearing Boschetto, we came upon an old bomb crater that had filled up with rainwater.

'Let's sit here, put our feet in the water, and have lunch,' suggested Eric. We had our swimming costumes on under our clothes, so we stripped off and settled down by the bomb crater. After the long walk, the cool of the water over our feet was bliss, and we sat there munching happily.

Eric had another idea. 'Let's jump in,' he said.

'You jump in first,' I said. 'See how deep it is.'

He plunged in without another word. 'Come in,' he called. 'It's splendid.'

Barbara and I dived into the water after him. It was gorgeous – so refreshing – like our own private swimming pool. The war and the hospital seemed a million miles away. We splashed around for a bit, and then I realised I was still wearing my wristwatch, a present from Auntie. It was gold, and quite precious. It had stopped.

Eric had a look. He opened it up and laid it in the sun to dry. 'If that doesn't bring any joy, I'll soak it in ether tonight.'

The sun treatment was of no use. So when we got back he collected a bottle of ether from the dispensary and left the watch in a shallow dish of the liquid. Though he knew little about mending watches he hoped this might clean it out and get it going again.

The following day I felt unwell. I assumed the walk had exhausted me, and was ashamed that I should have tired myself out on a jaunt when my duty was to the needs of the hospital and its patients. But it seemed more serious than simple fatigue. I was alarmed to think that it might even be the beginning of what Dr Chave-Cox had warned about. On the other hand, sand-fly fever was common in Malta, and it was possible I had succumbed to the viral infection these little moth-like midges could transmit. My temperature was certainly high, which is one of the symptoms. The normal treatment was to go to bed for a few days and recuperate. I would have insisted on such treatment if one of my patients had come down with sand-fly fever. But there could be no question of it for myself. I was the matron and I just had to work through it.

At the end of a long day, Eric came in after surgery and told me the ether hadn't worked. In my feverish state, I didn't quite know what he meant at first.

'Your watch,' he explained. 'It's still not going so I'm taking it to the menders now. They'll soon put it to rights.'

In the centre of Valletta, on the Strada Riale, under the Opera House, was a jeweller's. This was were Eric left the watch. He arranged to pick it up the following day.

That night there was a terrible raid. The Opera House was hit and totally destroyed. The next day when Eric went back, the jeweller's was no longer there. Nor, of course, was my watch.

April turned out to be the worst month of the blitz. Towards the end it seemed as if the enemy went all out to get us. One historian has written that Malta became the most bombed place on earth. More bombs were dropped on Malta than at the height of the Battle of Britain – a siege of annihilation.

When the onslaught was at its height, General Dobbie received this message from King George VI : 'To honour her brave people I award the George Cross to the Island Fortress of Malta to bear witness to a heroism and devotion that will long be famous in history.'

There continued to be heavy raids over the whole island, particularly centring on Mdina which had been

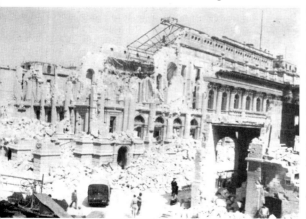

The Opera House destroyed

the ancient capital of Malta. It became known to us as the Silent City because the bells were stopped after bombs fell on all the churches there.

Nor was there any respite for us in Valletta. Bombs exploded with increasing ferocity around the Grand Harbour, shaking the hospital to its foundations; and one day even the heavy entrance doors were wrenched from their hinges in the blast and blown halfway down the main corridor.

Eric was walking down the corridor with the pharmacist, doing the rounds. I was making my way to join them when there was a sudden loud explosion outside and then a resounding din at the far end of the corridor as the doors crashed inwards and rattled towards us. The force of the explosion blew me off my feet and I went flying down the corridor as well. The doctor and the pharmacist saw me coming and opened their arms to catch me. The blast was so strong it forced all the air out of my body. Eric had to slap me and shake me to get me breathing again.

That night the bombs dropped more heavily still. This time they scored a direct hit on the hospital. We had managed to get into the shelter, and it was absolutely packed. The bombs exploded overhead. Everyone was scared stiff, they seemed so close. This time, I had to agree with our Maltese colleagues: it did seem like the end of the world. Once again, I got the nursing sisters to sing hymns with me to keep our spirits up.

By the time the air raid was over, the shelter was buried deep under rubble. Thankfully, General Dobbie's men were soon at hand and were eventually able to dig us out. When at last we emerged and saw the devastation the bombs had brought, we knew without doubt it was the end of KG5. In shock, some of the domestic staff picked up brooms and started sweeping the rubble from the corridors and off what remained of the stairs, but it was no good. Nothing was left standing. There were no beds. There were no walls. There were no facilities at all to treat the patients with. We could not continue to operate as a hospital.

The chef checked over what was left of the kitchen. When the sirens had sounded he had turned off the gas, but the large oven was still hot under a pile of rubble. Inside were large pans of rice he had put in for the evening meal. Amazingly, the rice was beautifully cooked and ready to be eaten. On top of the oven, intact, were large iron saucepans full of soup. Food for the patients and ourselves. Something warm and comforting to counteract the shock we were suffering. It was a kind of miracle.

We constructed makeshift tents out of bedsheets because, though it was not yet high summer, the heat of the midday sun could still be scorching. Eric arranged to have help sent over from Bighi, and they agreed to take in what patients they could. It was decided that we could transfer the more mobile to the hospital's recreational centre in Boschetto.

Everybody was safe. We had suffered no casualties. We had food and sustenance for our immediate needs. How we thanked the Lord for His saving grace, and for His goodness.

The date was the twenty-sixth of April. Primrose Day.

8

The Long Voyage Home

He ordered those who could swim to throw themselves overboard...
and so it was we all escaped
Acts 27.43-44

In time, we and our patients were relocated and we could at last return to a more settled regime of care for the sick and injured. The bombing eased over the next months. By July some advance by Allied forces had been made at sea. A great many mines were beginning to be cleared from Maltese waters. Ships were once again able to get into the Grand Harbour. As the year wore on, the Siege of Malta became the Relief of Malta.

Eric was worried about the condition of my health. He suspected I was suffering from delayed shock. General Dobbie had already left the island because of his health. He was replaced as governor by Field-Marshal Viscount Gort. Eric told him I should be sent home at the earliest opportunity.

The new governor promised to see what could be done. A few weeks later he informed us that a cargo ship which had managed to get into harbour a few nights before was just about to leave for England. He would see to it that I had a place on that ship. It was the *Clan Fraser* and was to set sail in convoy with another ship that had been waiting in harbour for safe passage.

A night or two before I was to leave, Eric took Barbara and me to dinner in one of the palaces. It was to be my farewell meal. After we had sat down and ordered, Eric took something out of his pocket and put it beside my plate. It was a small packet. 'What's that?' I asked him.

'Oh, just a little memento.'

It looked just about the size of a pen box.

'Can I open it and see what it is?'

He smiled. 'Yes, if you like.'

It was a watch – a tiny platinum wristwatch with an expanding bracelet strap. He leaned over and kissed me.

'I couldn't get a gold one,' he said. 'But this is the next best thing.'

Then Barbara handed me a package. It was a picture – a watercolour she had painted herself. It depicted Valletta harbour and the little Maltese fishing boats which in more peaceful days used to sail in and out by the score. She had given it the title *A Calm Dawn*.

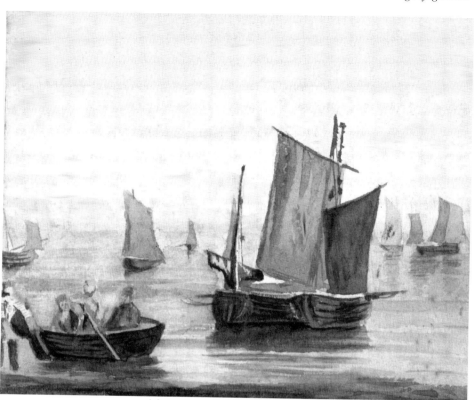

A Calm Dawn by Barbara Tyndale Biscoe

The day came for my departure. It was December 1942. Eric came down to the quayside to see me off. We introduced ourselves to the captain, and it was only then I discovered I was to be the only woman on board.

The captain's name was Giles. He told me that I had been allocated the pilot's cabin. It was next door to his cabin. There was no pilot on board. None would be needed until we reached Gibraltar. The captain warned me to have no illusions. It was true that the Axis powers no longer had complete control of the Mediterranean but it was going to be a dangerous crossing.

Eric handed two letters to Captain Giles. One, I knew, was for the ship's doctor, a Dr Shepherd, informing him of my condition and the results of Eric's tests on me. I did not know what the other letter was. Then we said our goodbyes and I went aboard. It had taken eight days to come out to Malta. The return journey was to take twenty-four. We would still be at sea on Christmas Day.

'I'll be thinking of you at Christmas,' promised Eric.

As we sailed out of the harbour I could see him standing with one of the sisters, Joanne, on the roof of the hospital, waving us goodbye. It was with great sadness that I left Malta.

Once on board I was made most welcome, but the captain apologised when he told me I would have to wear a life jacket over my ordinary clothes. 'I'm afraid I must ask you to keep that on at all times,' he said. 'Even at night when you're asleep.'

There was a twinkle in his eye as he said this – in fact, I was often unsure whether he was teasing me or not about some things – but I saw that none of the crew were without their life jackets and it brought home to me how we could never consider ourselves safe until we reached our destination.

Captain Giles must have been in his late fifties, but he still had a full head of dark hair. He was clean-shaven and about six foot tall. He told me his friends called him Gilo and that I must do the same. He looked after me well, making sure that I was comfortable. He had an Indian lascar who was to see I had all I needed. I was to take all my meals with the captain. After having so little in Malta it was glorious to have good food again. Occasionally Dr Shepherd might have coffee with us, but the captain would not allow any of the crew to join us. Since I was the only woman on the ship he gave orders that no one else was to fraternise with me.

Dr Shepherd and I had met before. He had been a dinner party guest at my aunt's house. It happened to be on one of her Remembrance Day birthday dinners. In the middle of the table she had set out an arrangement of poppies. They cascaded down, spilling over on to the white tablecloth, like blood on snow, in honour of the men who had lost their lives in the Great War. She had recently met Dr Shepherd, who at that time had been an osteopath, and had invited him along. She was having some treatment from him. What a coincidence it was that we should meet again in the middle of another terrible war.

Dr Shepherd was middle-aged and tubby, and his manner was rather ingratiating. I wasn't sure I liked him. It was as if, because of our acquaintance through Auntie, he felt he had some claim over me and he tried to play on this. Quite early on he asked me, 'Have you brought any mementos back with you?'

'Yes,' I said, 'I have. Just little things to remind me of my time at KG5. I bought a set of dinner mats for Auntie and for my sister Mary. Oh, and a couple of tablecloths.'

'I came away in such a hurry I didn't manage to get anything like that,' he said. 'You wouldn't be able to spare me something, would you? I'd pay you, of course.'

For someone I did not know terribly well it seemed a rather forward request, but since I did have one or two extra bits and pieces I felt I should oblige. I never said anything to the captain, but he must have been aware of my unease because after a while Dr Shepherd was no longer encouraged to take coffee with us.

We had embarked on the most momentous journey. The war at sea was now at its height. German submarines and bombers were still inflicting terrible damage on our Allied shipping. The raiders were soon to be heard overhead – Italian and German planes, measuring up their targets. We travelled without convoy, unescorted by battleships, and we were camouflaged in certain ways I didn't quite understand, but it seemed to put the enemy off our trail. They appeared to be more interested in other vessels that would come into view.

It was alarming to see, out on the horizon, the ships they had chosen to attack, burning and sinking under plumes of smoke. We would watch helplessly as a sheaf of bombs dropped from a plane, or a U-boat surfaced and sent a torpedo speeding towards its target. The ship would be engulfed in flames, and in a matter of minutes it would sink and completely disappear under the sea. We counted ourselves fortunate but were sad for those unlucky enough to be hit.

Heading towards Gibraltar we had to pass through the mined waters of Palmeira. Occasionally depth charges would explode around us. One night I thought we were under attack as I heard the muffled explosions of disturbed mines or detonated depth charges. It was just as if our ship had been hit. I was fearful, but I knew the Lord was with me. The message which I had taken with me to Malta, and which carried me through my time there, was giving me comfort now on my way home. And I knew many people would be praying for us.

It was nevertheless a frightening time for us all. Gilo attempted to comfort me. 'Come on, now,' he would say. 'Don't worry about these bombings. We'll be all right.'

To keep exercised Gilo used to walk six times round the decks, twice a day. He said I was to walk with him. 'It'll keep your legs firm and get some fresh air into those lungs.' When we got to the prow, he would start singing. He had a fine baritone voice. He would sing all the old songs – *Don't Go Down the Mines, Dad* and *Down the Vale* and *The Great Divide*. As his voice rolled out over the waters it brought back to mind our family get-togethers with my father singing at the piano.

One Sunday morning Gilo invited the captain from our companion ship, and some of his officers and midshipmen, to join us for coffee. It was a great pleasure to meet all these brave men. They told me that when they had come under Gilo's command he had given each of them a copy of Kipling's *If*. They had a few days only to learn it by heart and be able repeat it to him. He believed that this built up their confidence. I also discovered that one of the officers was engaged to Gilo's daughter.

Two days later there was another heavy bombardment. Our companion ship was hit, and some of those young men whom I had met that day were killed – including the captain's prospective son-in-law.

Soon after this we received information that one of the U-boats responsible for the attack had been depth-charged and was breaking up. The *Clan Fraser* was to keep a look-out for any survivors who might be clinging to the wreckage in the water, and stand by to pick them up. I was on the bridge with the captain when some survivors were spotted. 'Oh,' I said, 'that's good.'

'What's good about it?' asked the captain.

'Well, they haven't all perished. We'll be able to save some of them. And I'll be able to help the doctor see to their needs when you bring them on board.'

Gilo took me to one side. He was extremely upset and angry. 'You're not doing anything of the sort. You're a civilian on this ship. You're not going to soil your fingers by so much as touching those filthy Germans.'

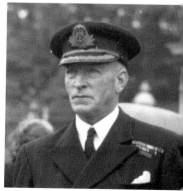

Captain Giles

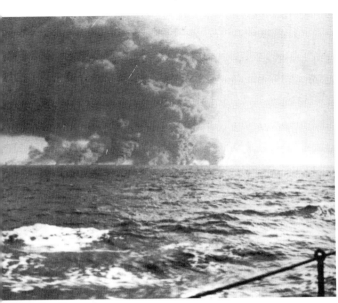

Searching for survivors

'But I'm a nurse. I'm neutral. I must do what I can to help them. If they've been in the water any length of time they'll be suffering from exposure. They'll need proper medical care. Dr Shepherd can't look after them all on his own. Please, I must help.'

'You're not touching them,' he repeated. 'Besides, it might be one of their dirty tricks. They can make it look as though they've broken up. They release clothing and other flotsam from their U-boats. That way they slow us down, make us sitting targets.'

I knew why he was so upset: it was because of his daughter's fiancé. But it did not prepare me for what he was about to say.

'You met those fine young men of ours. And now they're gone. They lost their lives because of the Hun down there. We're not picking them up. We're going on. We're keeping full steam ahead.'

I was shocked that he could do such a cold-blooded thing. But I realised that this was the terrible reality of war. He was a good man. For those few long weeks at sea he had been like a father to me. But now it was a war captain who stood before me. I saw it was no use arguing with him any further.

When we arrived at Gibraltar, Gilo came to my cabin. 'Mina, I want you to come up on deck,' he said. Once we had got up there he asked, 'Now what do you see?'

At first I thought it was a great grey rock. As we got closer I saw it was a ship: 'A big black ship,' I said, 'like a huge dark wall on the sea.'

'Yes. It's an aircraft carrier. The *Ark Royal*. You've heard of the *Ark Royal*, haven't you?' He pointed towards the top of the 'wall'. 'Look right up there. There's a kind of tower. Can you see a platform?'

I wasn't sure. I could see a sailor with two flags. He was waving them about.

'He's doing semaphore,' Gilo explained. 'He's sending a message.'

There was a sudden loud roar. An aeroplane shot into view from behind the 'wall'. It was closely followed by another. They must have been taking off from the deck, high above where we stood.

'What else can you see?' demanded the captain.

'Well, there are a lot of men standing all along the edge of the wall. Are they standing on the deck?'

'Yes. Those are all the *Ark Royal's* officers and sailors. Now if you look right up there on the tower, you'll see a little door open. There's a platform there, and shortly an officer will come out and stand on that platform.'

As I watched I saw an opening in the turret of the ship and an officer stepped out. Gilo handed me a pair of binoculars. Now I could see that the officer had gold braid and a row of medals on his chest.

'That's the Admiral of the Fleet, Lord Cunningham,' said Gilo. 'And he's giving a message which will be transcribed by that sailor.'

The sailor started waving the flags again.

'Now, let me see, what is the Admiral's message?' he muttered as he took back the binoculars and trained them on the flag-waver. 'He's congratulating you on being the first woman to pass through the mined waters of the Palmeira. He's wishing you well on your home journey. He's asking the men of the *Ark Royal* to give three cheers for the lady.'

Suddenly all the men lined up on the deck cheered three times, and waved their hands. I felt sure that Gilo was having me on. He was forever teasing me about this and that. But his timing had been good. He had made it seem almost convincing.

'Don't be silly. They wouldn't put on all that show for me. I don't believe it.'

'Well, you may or may not believe it, but that's what the message said, and that's what they are honouring you for. You can watch me log it, if you like. Then perhaps you'll realise I'm telling you the truth.'

I stood by Gilo as he wrote in the log book:

> The Admiral of the Fleet today
> conveyed his congratulations to Mina
> Staerck, first woman to pass through
> these enemy waters. He wishes her
> well on her journey home.

Soon after that it was Christmas, which we were to spend moored off Gibraltar. We set out on the second leg of our journey only after the celebrations were over. On Christmas morning Gilo handed me an envelope.

'This is for you. Dr Doyle gave it to me the morning we left Malta – with strict instructions I was to hand it to you on Christmas Day and not before. Now you sit quietly somewhere and open it.'

So that's what the second envelope had been. How sweet of Eric to think so far ahead, I thought. It was such a touching gesture.

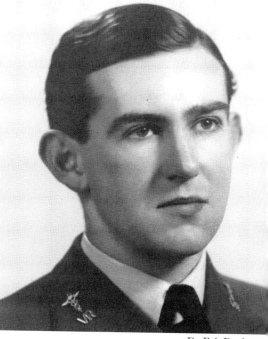

Dr Eric Doyle

I did exactly as the captain suggested. I found a quiet corner and opened the envelope. Inside was a simple little note wishing me a happy Christmas, hoping I was still well and assuring me how much he would be missing me on this of all days. I must admit I shed a tear or two. He had been such a good friend. I remembered all we had been through together and prayed that he was safe and sound in Malta. I thought of all those on Malta and prayed that they would have a happy day this Christmas, free of raids. I thought of all my loved ones at home. I thanked the Lord for bringing us safe so far, through that dangerous stretch of sea. I felt sure He would be with us to our journey's end.

That night the captain and I were to have a full Christmas dinner. In my baggage I had packed away an evening dress which I had hardly worn since coming out to Malta. I put it on to make it a really special occasion. 'It's in your honour,' I told him.

It was a delightful meal. The first officer was allowed to join us for coffee.

Though we were berthed at Gibraltar for some days, we were not allowed to leave the ship. One day Dr Shepherd said to me, 'You've been cooped up on board long enough. I'm going ashore for lunch. Why not come with me? There's a fine place here. It's called the Bristol Hotel.'

'Can we?' I asked.

'Yes, of course,' he answered. 'I've asked them to lower a boat for us.'

Because we were anchored in the deeper waters of the bay – alongside the *Ark Royal* – we had to be ferried across from the ship. Naturally, I thought he had permission from the captain. When we got ashore we had to pass through customs. They were most suspicious. Dr Shepherd had no passport. Nor did I. Our reasons for coming ashore sounded pretty feeble in answer to their stern questions. Finally, and grudgingly, they allowed us through. The doctor led me along the narrow harbour streets until we came to the Bristol Hotel.

We had just sat down and were about to order lunch when the doctor was called outside by Gibraltar police. I could hear their low serious voices but caught nothing of what they said. When he came back he looked pale.

'Come on, Mina. We've got to go somewhere with these gentlemen.'

I got up and followed him. To my horror we soon found ourselves locked up in jail.

'Why have they put us in here?' I asked him.

'Because we haven't got our papers with us.'

'Did you let the captain know about our trip ashore?' He didn't reply at once, and I began to feel worried. I repeated my question. 'Did you ask the captain for permission?'

'Oh, it's all right. He won't mind us coming across.'

My worry was growing. 'Well, you'll have to tell him we're here. Ask them to ring the *Clan Fraser* and get the captain to vouch for us.' But Dr Shepherd was the kind of man who had an answer for everything.

'Oh, it'll be enough to have told them who we are. They'll get in touch with the captain.'

That's what happened. Eventually. Gilo had to send his first officer across with our identification. At last, we were free to go.

'You're in for it. The captain's furious with you,' said the first officer as we stood behind him in the little boat on the journey back to the ship. Then he turned to me and added, 'Not with you, Miss Staerck,' and nodded towards the doctor. 'Not with you, but with him.'

Back in the captain's cabin, Gilo seemed to be no less furious with me, after he had given the doctor a dressing down and dismissed him.

'Why on earth did you go?' he shouted.

'I thought Dr Shepherd had got your permission,' I protested.

'Thought? You know what thought did. I knew nothing about it. You realise you might have been jailed for life?'

I never really considered that a serious possibility. Was the captain teasing me again? It was difficult to be certain.

On leaving Gibraltar we had to steal out under the cover of night, heavily camouflaged. There was no knowing where the enemy was and when we might be singled out for attack. There were spies and informants everywhere. It was imperative that every precaution be taken, if we were to reach England in one piece. But in the end it was not a human enemy that was to test us to the limit.

A terrific storm broke out. It became so bad that we had difficulty standing and walking. Things were sliding about dangerously. Everything had to be secured: tables and chairs were bolted to the floor; cargo and supplies were roped up; even I was strapped into my bunk with special straps that the captain's lascar pulled tight so that I would not fall out and injure myself. That night I made sure I was wearing my life jacket.

The ship was buffeted from all sides and rolled alarmingly this way and that in the huge waves. I could hear them crashing on to the decks above. But I knew the Lord was in the whirlwind and the storm. He had promised that He would go before, and I put my trust in Him.

Despite the commotion I must have fallen into a deep sleep, because the next thing I knew the spray was drenching me. The captain and the first officer were either side of me, supporting me, as we made for the stern. The waves were rising higher than the ship – thirty or forty feet high – and crashing over us. The deck was at an ever-changing angle, as the ship lurched this way and that. Every step was a battle. Eventually we reached the rail.

'Get up on here,' the captain ordered. 'Sit on this rail.'

I must have looked horror-stricken.

'Don't worry,' he shouted through the storm. 'I'll hold on to you. You won't fall. The first officer will hold you on the other side. Now, we're going to jump together. When I say jump, you must jump.'

There were, I saw now, several other members of the crew clambering over the rails and jumping into the darkness below.

'Oh, I can't!' I said, the terror rising in me.

'You must! You see down there, there's a lifeboat. That's what we're aiming for.'

Looking down into the dark waters I could just make out the lifeboat. Some of the crew were already in it. They were stretching a blanket between them, trying to catch the men as they went crashing down and break their fall. The idea that I should follow their example filled me with horror. I felt I couldn't possibly jump.

'Just push your feet against the rail and let yourself go. The men in the boat will try to catch you. If you miss the boat and go into the water, hold your breath, and when you surface grab anything you can. They'll do their best to pick you up.'

Still I held back. I was too afraid to jump.

'The ship's going down, Mina,' the captain said. 'Either way, you'll end up in the water. Its cold, and you won't last long. Ten minutes at the most.'

If ever I was near the brink of death, it seemed I was then. The captain put his arm round me and put his mouth to my ear. 'I'd hoped to see you back to the Clyde. Pray God we'll get there still. So, Mina – jump!'

I jumped. It was all like a dream. Water closed over my head. The next I knew the captain was shouting at me. 'Kick off your shoes, Mina. Kick off your shoes!'

I must have missed the boat. Somehow I had managed to get hold of a plank of wood or something. They must have jumped as well. Between them, Gilo and the first officer were supporting me in the water. 'Hang on to it, Mina! Hang on!' they yelled. They were swimming either side of me, pulling me towards the boat. The men in the lifeboat leaned over us and threw a kind of net down. We grabbed on to it and they hauled us up. I don't remember much after that. As they led me to one end of the boat and sat me down, I remember being thankful there was something solid beneath my feet again, even if it was the rocking boat. I remember that my feet were cold, and my clothes were wringing wet. And then from somewhere brandy was produced. After that I can remember nothing at all.

The *Clan Fraser* did not go under. We were picked up by the other ship and when the storm had abated were able to go back to our own. A few days later we arrived in the Clyde.

We were held up for five days in Loch Long. Captain Giles told me that he had received a message from the harbour authorities. He was expecting visitors.

'What's happening?' I asked Gilo.

'The message I had was from the War Office,' he replied gravely. 'We have a fifth-columnist on board.'

A boatful of military police boarded the ship and after a brief search they led a man away. I was astounded to discover it was Dr Shepherd. The captain reminded me that the doctor had written numerous postcards. When his medical reports were taken ashore he had the cards sent too. It turned out he had been writing in code, disclosing information about the ship, its route and destination. He had told the captain that he had a number of nieces and nephews who would be interested to hear from him. We thought him a dutiful uncle. In fact, he was a traitor.

It was at first difficult to grasp fully the calculated callousness of what he had done. Gradually it began to sink in. I kept going over my conversations with him. Had I given anything vital away? But the worst realisation was that he may even have been responsible for the attack on our companion ship, in which the fiancé of Gilo's daughter had been killed.

Now we were allowed to go ashore ourselves. Gilo and I were met by his wife Dorothy and his two daughters. The captain turned to me.

'During this difficult voyage, Mina,' he said, 'I've looked upon you as if you were another of my daughters. Now you must come and stay with us at our hotel until you can arrange to get to London.'

We travelled to Edinburgh. At the hotel I was able to make a phone call to Auntie. I wasn't able to speak to her direct but I left messages to say I would be coming home in a day or two. I stayed the night at the hotel and got to know Gilo's family. They were so kind to me. Despite my protests, the captain paid for my room and next day booked my London sleeper.

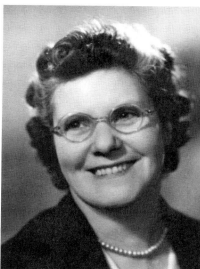

I shall never forget that journey – I mean the one from Edinburgh to London. Glad as I was to be off the ship, and on my way to London again, those eight hours seemed to take an eternity. The train was cold and noisy, and the bunk was narrower and harder than the one on the ship. I didn't sleep a wink.

My sister Mary and her husband Frank were there at Kings Cross to meet me. I kissed and hugged them both. It was so nice to see them.

My sister Mary, and below, her husband Frank Goldsmith making a violin

'Where's Auntie?' I asked. I was surprised not to see her on the platform. I was longing to tell her all about my time in Malta.

'She couldn't come, Mina,' said Mary. 'She asked if we would meet you in. She's had to move from that big house of hers in St John's Wood.'

'Why?'

'They're pulling down that row,' explained Frank. 'A lot of them are unsafe because of the bombing. They're making them into mansion flats.'

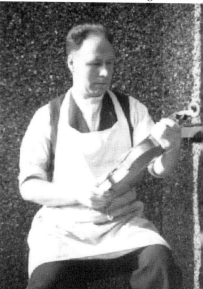

'But she's made arrangements for you to stay at Finchley Road,' added Mary. This was a home for missionaries Auntie helped run.

I was upset not to be able to see Auntie straightaway after all I had been through. But at least I was back home. Safe and sound.

9

Barnardo's

Let the children come to me, and do not hinder them;
for to such belongs the kingdom of heaven
Matthew 19.14

Because of Dr Eric Doyle's concern about my medical condition, I had to go to Dr Chave-Cox for another examination. This time he had something specific and apparently serious to report. According to him I had endocarditis – inflammation of the heart. I was not even to think of working for at least the next six months.

Auntie Dagmar's new home was Welbeck House in Hove and she kindly took me down there to live with her again while I followed the doctor's advice and tried to rest. But Britain was still at war and my aunt was as lively as ever. As a result, rest was not always easy to come by. Though the worst of the Blitz was over and the air raids were few and far between compared to what I had experienced in Malta and on the voyage home, London remained a dangerous place to be. But even in Hove we were not completely out of danger. Doodlebugs – the unpiloted flying bombs – were still being sent over from Germany. We would sometimes hear them pass overhead, and not all of them would have the fuel in their rockets to take them to their destination. It was always possible that they might drop down on us.

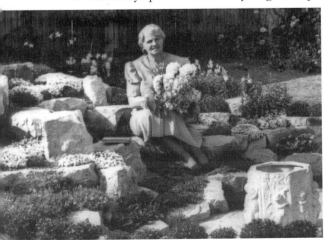

Auntie had excavated a bomb shelter in the foundations of the house. She had put up curtains all round the walls to hide the bricks, and put in a couple of bunks. When the sirens sounded we used to take a book to read or some knitting. There was a little stove and some supplies down there so we could make a meal if the all-clear signal was a long time coming. It was really rather cozy. Fortunately, Auntie's house was never hit.

Auntie in the rock garden at Welbeck House in Hove

All this time, unbeknown to me, Barnardo's had been trying to contact me. They knew I had a connection with the CIM, so eventually they applied to the mission for help in locating me. One week Auntie happened to go to one of their prayer meetings, which were still held in Stoke Newington. At the end of the meeting one of the elders came up to her and started to chat.

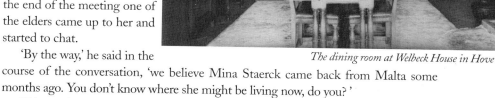

The dining room at Welbeck House in Hove

'By the way,' he said in the course of the conversation, 'we believe Mina Staerck came back from Malta some months ago. You don't know where she might be living now, do you?'

'Oh, yes,' replied Auntie. 'She's with me.'

'Really?' said the elder. 'What a coincidence! We've been trying to find her for weeks. Barnardo's have been asking for her.'

'She's got to rest for six months on doctor's orders,' Auntie told him. 'The siege in Malta has taken it out of her, poor girl.'

'Well, now that we know her whereabouts, we'll pass on her address to Barnardo's, if we may. She'll be getting a letter from them shortly.'

'I don't know if it'll be of much use. She can't start working for them for a while yet, if that's what they want.'

But the letter duly arrived. It was to say that they were looking for a matron for the hospital at Boys' Garden City in Woodford Bridge. Miss Phillips, the old matron, had finally retired and it was her wish that I be contacted. She had put forward my name as her successor. If I wanted to apply for the job, I would be considered along with the other applicants. They gave a time and date for me to have an interview with them at their headquarters in Stepney Causeway.

Remembering the way in which those stamps had turned up for my letter of application all those years ago, and Miss Phillips' kind words and her extraordinary suggestion that I should one day succeed her as matron, it seemed wrong to turn my back on this opportunity. I had rested for a month or so, and was feeling much recovered, so with mounting excitement at the prospect I attended the interview and got the job. I was appointed matron of the Capel Hanbury Hospital. It was to be my longest engagement yet.

Boys' Garden City had been purpose-built as a self-contained community. It was modelled on Letchworth and Welwyn Garden City which were built from scratch early this century to relieve the terrible congestion and overcrowding of industrial cities like London. They were designed to provide a mix of country

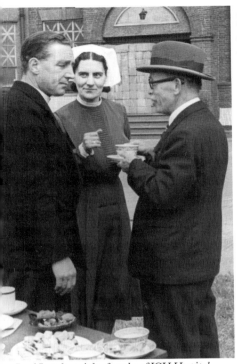

Lord Lyttelton right, founder of JCH Hospital

living and town life, being surrounded by countryside and yet having all the facilities a town might offer.

The John Capel Hanbury Hospital was part of this self-contained community. It had been founded by Lord Lyttelton on whose land the 'City' was built on. He had given the hospital its name.

Within the grounds was a fully-equipped school and a beautiful little church, a gymnasium and an indoor swimming pool, and a large assembly hall for prayers and entertainments and speech-days. The living quarters for the boys were made up of a number of separate houses. In each house about twenty boys of all ages were looked after by a 'father' and a 'mother'. The voluntary positions of 'aunts' and 'uncles' were filled by people from the neighbouring districts who would visit on a regular basis and become involved with the children as a kind of extended family. They would organise trips and give presents at birthdays and Christmas.

A separate building of about a hundred rooms provided accommodation for the nurses and staff. Then there was the house in which the governor of the home lived. His name was Mr Cobbald.

Near to the Boys' Garden City was a mental hospital. Its grounds were adjacent to ours. We could see the men in various states of disturbance walking about and we were worried lest any of the more dangerous patients wandered into our grounds. We had to be alert, but I'm glad to say there were no incidents while I was there.

Winston Churchill was the MP for the Woodford Bridge area. When I started as matron he was the prime minister and still busy winning the war for us, so we didn't see anything of him, but Lady Churchill did come once and present prizes at our speech day.

I was given the task of finding out what she would be wearing, so that they could choose appropriate colours for the bouquet that was going to be given to her. They didn't want anything that might clash. I rang Downing Street from the governor's house and I asked what time exactly she would be arriving and if anything special might be required for her. Then I asked how she would be dressed. It was going to be a 'floral design', I was informed, of 'autumnal colouring'. With some trepidation, we ordered a large arrangement of chrysanthemums. Happily, on the day she and they were a perfect match.

She made her address and presented the trophies and prizes and then visited the various houses. Her visit was tremendously popular with the boys since a grand tea was laid on for her, and they could all tuck in as well!

Several years later, after the war was over, he did come and see us once for a quick visit with the governor, but he didn't come to look round the hospital.

Auntie Dagmar used to come for the speech days, too. She would travel from Hove in one of her big cars. The first year, she parked it in front of one of the boys' houses. It aroused a great deal of interest. When we came outside again, the car was covered with them: boys of every size, climbing all over it and sitting on the roof and bonnet.

I called Mr Cresswell, the caretaker, and one or two of the other men, and they managed to clear Auntie's car for her. Surprisingly, she took it very well. In fact she found it rather amusing. I think she realised the boys had meant no harm. They were simply curious and excited at seeing such a magnificent and rare spectacle in the grounds of their own home.

Despite this incident, Auntie came up to see me quite often. The matron's quarters were comfortable, and perfect for entertaining visitors as well as dealing with official matters. There was a large lounge with a fine grand piano. For relaxation I practised on it, trying to relearn some lost skills. And in the corner were two elegant high-backed chairs with low, delicately cane-woven seats. Miss Phillips had kindly left them for me.

Off the lounge was an office where I could get on with the administrative duties on which Miss Phillips had laid such emphasis all those years before. Luckily I was provided with a secretary, which was a great help.

London was not far away. Coming from the city centre one could get a tube to Woodford, and from there it was a twenty minute walk or a short bus ride. In Woodford Bridge I was only a mile or so from Leytonstone where I had lived with my cousins Edith and Hilda, and later, my brother Eddie, and had gone to school in Mayville Road.

Dr Barnardo's first home – in East London – was called simply the Boys' Home and was set up in 1870 for the care of homeless and destitute children, mainly boys. Then in 1876 he founded the Girls' Village Home in Barkingside. This was only just down the road from Woodford Bridge. We shared a medical superintendent, a senior doctor named Gilmore.

Our own consultant physician was a nice man called Milne. He was only four foot six – what we would now called a person of restricted growth. Imagine my surprise when I discovered that his sister was the same Miss Milne that had been matron of St Mary's, Paddington, when I had taken my exams. Miss Milne and I soon met up again, both of us matrons now, and became firm friends.

Dr Milne's family connections did not stop there, for his brother was a famous orthopaedic surgeon of the time, and he would come and operate for us, entirely free of charge. Over these years changes were taking place in Britain which meant that charity was not for much longer going to be the only hope of those who could not afford to pay for good health and education. In 1942 the Beveridge Report had looked into the feasibility of a new idea – free health provision for everyone. But the NHS was a few years away yet and the charitable commitment made by Dr Milne's brother, and several other London consultants who were happy to come and give their services free, was at that time tremendously important for our work.

I'm proud to say that the level of health care we provided at Capel Hanbury was high, and it soon occurred to me that we should establish a training school at the hospital. I contacted the General Nursing Council and floated the idea of teaching the nursing of sick children. Boys' Garden City seemed the ideal place to do it.

The matron of Guy's Hospital, Miss McManus, and my friend Miss Milne – who was still matron of St Mary's – both came to assess the possibility. They read my report and agreed that even if it was not possible to set up a full training school on the site, it should at least become affiliated with other hospitals in the teaching of nurses, and that it could provide an ideal training ground for the treatment of sick children.

It took another two years of writing reports, attending meetings and so on before the affiliation was set up. In the reorganisation that the National Health Service would soon bring, England was to be divided into fourteen regions. Each Regional Health Authority was to have at least one medical school and teaching hospital, and from 1945 the John Capel Hanbury Hospital was finally recognised as a Preliminary Training School (or PTS) by the General Nursing Council. Nurses would come for their first two years of training, and then go on to one of the larger affiliated hospitals, King Edward Memorial Hospital, Ealing, or the Connaught Hospital in Walthamstow.

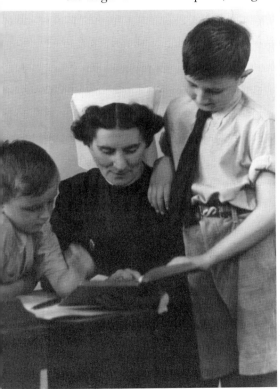

There were some lovely boys at JCH

The children taken in by Barnardo's were no longer predominantly waifs and strays. Increasingly, the 'orphans' were the result of divorces, or of the deaths caused by the war. I met some lovely boys at JCH. They would sometimes sing to me. *Waltzing Matilda* was a particular favourite of mine.

In those days Barnardo's used to send parties of boys out to Australia, accompanied by a member of the Barnardo's Council. Prospects were thought to be better over there, away from the squalor and deprivation of the city life in Britain. Arrangements would first be made – that two dozen boys, say, could be found a certain job, or be trained for one, or be apprenticed in some trade such as farm work or building. Sometimes an old boy would turn up out of the blue on a trip back to the old country. Australia would often mark a change of fortune for them and several who called in on us had become quite prosperous.

In England, the Watt's Naval school would take in any Barnardo's boy who was old enough and had an interest in sailing. They would receive a nautical training which might equip them to become merchant seamen or take up service in the Royal Navy.

As matron I was supplied with a maid, as well as a secretary: Barnardo's had a place where they trained their own girls for domestic service. To give them work experience and to provide the homes with reliable staff, HQ would send these girls to various Barnardo's homes around the country. Over the time I was there I had three different girls. They were all good at their job, and I became very fond of them.

One day, as I was dictating a letter to my secretary, the first of my girls, whose name was Jean, knocked on my office door.

'Matron, there's a visitor for you.'

'Oh, yes? Who's that?'

'I don't rightly know, matron. He wouldn't give his name. But he wants to see you.'

'Well, sit him in my lounge, make him some coffee and ask him if he'll wait for a few minutes. I'm in conference at the moment.'

'All right, matron.'

My dictation took a little longer than anticipated. When I finished I remembered that there was a visitor waiting. I walked into the lounge. My heart leapt! It was Eric Doyle.

'Mina. How good to see you,' he said, and he took me in his arms and kissed me.

'When did you get back?' I asked him.

'I've only just got back this moment,' he replied.

He had stayed in Malta for another two years. The King George V Hospital had been rebuilt and the work of caring for patients – war-wounded and otherwise – had gone on regardless. Malta's part in the war was now virtually over. Eric had at last been free to leave.

'It's all been rather hurried,' he added. 'I've not been over to Ireland yet, so I've not even seen my mother. But while I was passing through London I did want to make sure you were OK. The CIM told me you were here. It's my first port of call.'

I was flattered, and of course overjoyed to see him.

While we were chatting away and drinking our coffee, a messenger came to say that Dr Milne had fallen and hurt himself. Could we get a doctor to see to him?

I tried contacting our medical superintendent at Barkingside but could not get hold of him. I turned to Eric. 'I know it's an imposition,' I said,' but would you mind going along and seeing how badly hurt Dr Milne is?'

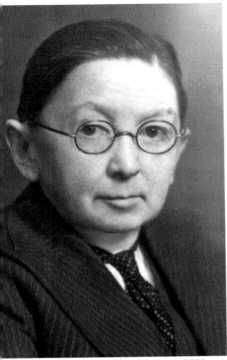

Dr James Milne, consultant physician to JCH

'Of course I will,' he answered at once and went off straightaway with the messenger. When he came back, the news was not good.

'He's broken his leg,' he said. 'It's rather serious.'

After the incident was over, and Dr Milne had been transported to the nearest casualty department, there was little time left to spend with Eric. He had to get back to London and then take a boat over to Ireland. It had been a wonderful reunion, if much too brief.

In addition to the maid, HQ sent a couple of severely handicapped teenage girls who had been trained in professional seamstressing and general sewing work at one of the other Barnardo's Homes. I was glad to take them in, and accommodated them in one of the side wards of the hospital. They could look after themselves quite happily and they met all the sewing needs of the hospital. They were no trouble whatsoever and I was pleased with their work. They were performing a useful job, which was good for them as well as us. I believe they enjoyed being with us, and they certainly appreciated being gainfully employed. But it was because of them that I eventually had to leave Barnardo's.

It came to our attention that the head superintendent of Barnardo's was giving up the post and that the position was being taken up by a Mr Lucette. One day, Mr Lucette came on a visit to the Boys' Garden City.

When he was introduced to our two seamstresses, he wanted to know what they were doing there. He seemed to find it hard to believe our perfectly truthful explanation – that they were holding down a useful job. He thought they were there under false pretences, that Barnardo's charitable resources were being misdirected. What he actually said was, 'Barnardo's cannot afford to have passengers'.

I was incensed. 'They're not passengers,' I said. 'They're earning their keep.'

'Well, never mind,' he persisted. 'They must go back to where they came from.'

I refused point-blank to agree to this shameful demand, and Mr Lucette appeared to give way in the face of my determined stance. But a few days later, knowing me to be away on business, he called again and made arrangements in my absence for the girls to be picked up and sent back to their original Home.

When I discovered what had happened I realised my autonomy as matron had been compromised. So strongly did I feel about it that I wrote immediately to Mr Kirkpatrick, the previous head superintendent, and to Dr Gilmore, the medical superintendent, stating my feelings about the issue and informing them that I was tendering my resignation. I asked them both for references.

Dr Gilmore came to see me. He was upset that I was leaving. But I said, 'It's no good, I can't look after this hospital if Mr Lucette is going to step in and override my authority.'

That Tuesday, as every Tuesday, there was a committee meeting of the Barnardo's managers. Mr Kirkpatrick and several others from headquarters came down. I gave my hospital report as usual and then explained why I felt it

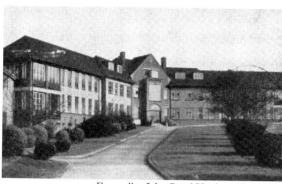

Farewell to John Capel Hanbury Hospital

necessary to resign. The committee members expressed their regret and tried to persuade me to stay. But my decision was made. Each of them wrote to me afterwards saying how sad they were to see me go.

It was 1948. I had been matron of Barnardo's for six years and for all of that time had received £120 per year. This was on the low side even then – but Barnardo's was a charity and I did have my accommodation and meals provided. Besides, my earnings as a nurse had always been meagre. The first substantial increase in salary during my years in nursing was as matron at the Kent and Sussex Hospital, which was my next appointment. The rise resulted from the report on nurses' earnings by the Rushcliffe Committee which was part and parcel of the introduction that year of the National Health Service.

From the Kent and Sussex I moved on to Beckenham, Kent, as a tutor and home sister in the local hospital. My friend, Kay Wilson, knew the matron of Beckenham, who had suddenly lost her tutor. Kay suggested that I might be interested in filling in while she sorted things out on a more permanent basis. The matron's name was Belle Houston. I agreed to help her out for a month.

It was a nice little hospital. The accommodation was good and I liked the set-up of the teaching classrooms. Though I had not formally taught nurses before, it seemed to come naturally and was something I thoroughly enjoyed. Soon the month was up, but there was still no word of a replacement.

At the time, the Ministry of Health happened to be circulating a paper advertising an extra-mural course in nurse training – resulting in a sister tutor diploma. It was 1949, and with the expansion of the hospital services for the NHS, the Ministry needed to train many more nurses. The two-year full-time course was being offered by King's College London and the London College of Nursing. Full salary would be payable over the whole period.

I had the qualifications and nursing experience required for the tutor's diploma. The teaching of nurses was the route I felt my career should be taking and I felt it was time to think about moving on from Beckenham: I had already been there longer than anticipated. By the time I applied for the course all the places had been filled. I was informed that King's College was running an external course at Hull University. I should apply to them.

I wrote off straightaway, and the application forms duly arrived for me to complete. The consent and signature of the matron for whom I was working was required. I went to Belle with the form and told her what I was planning to do.

'Oh, you can't go,' she said.

'Why on earth not?'

'Well, I'll be left without a tutor again.'

'But I only agreed to come here for a month,' I said, 'and I've been here nearly two.'

'Well,' said Belle, 'I'm not letting you go.'

I felt she was treating me unfairly, so I went to see the London College of Nursing, and also the General Nursing Council. Both knew me well, for by this time I was on the Board of Examiners to the General Council and had had extensive dealings with both institutions as matron at Barnardo's. Each of them gave me assurances that Belle Houston could not stop me taking up the diploma course, and each wrote to the Beckenham Hospital Management Committee authorising my departure.

Did I but know it, I was not only leaving Beckenham Hospital. I was saying goodbye to one kind of life, and embarking on an altogether different one.

10

The Man Upstairs

In Him we live and move and have our being
Acts 17.28

When I came to Hull for the interview at the university it was the first time I had visited the city. It was raining and terribly cold. I thought what a ugly place it was. Everywhere seemed to be boarded up. The city had been heavily bombed during the war.

I was accepted for the course. Next, I had to find somewhere to live.

Bob Hutchinson was a worker at Auntie's mission, an accountant who later was to inch his way into her financial affairs. He knew a gentleman in Hull, a Christian called Mr Priestman, who might introduce me to a church there and also have some ideas about accommodation. He wrote to him at once.

A letter duly arrived from Mr Priestman. He informed me that he had just taken over a house in Hull. The ground floor flat was to be vacated by the present occupier, a headmistress who was taking up missionary work in India. If I liked I could rent the flat. There was a Christian gentleman living upstairs who would arrange things for me. The only problem was that the day I was due to start at the university was three weeks before the date the headmistress was to leave. However, Mr Priestman said that there was a nearby guest house, the Dorchester, which could put me up.

Term began on the fourth of October. I started packing, looking forward with mixed feelings to the year I was to spend in Hull.

On my arrival at the Dorchester Guest House I was handed a letter of welcome from the headmistress – a Miss Marjorie Beevers – and some flowers she had kindly left for my room. The letter invited me to come and look round the flat at any time.

Number Five Eldon Grove, where Miss Beevers lived, was literally just around the corner in a private cul-de-sac of large Victorian town houses which ran alongside the Dorchester. The next morning I went straight round to see where I would be living while studying at the university.

The flat seemed so big. It had sounded marvellous from Mr Priestman's description in his letter, but it had large dingy rooms,

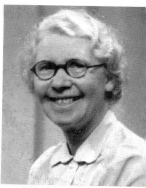

Miss Marjorie Beevers

high ceilings and felt cold and damp. Though I didn't say anything to Miss Beevers, I came away thinking that I'd never be able to look after myself and the flat, and do my studying as well. I decided to write to Mr Priestman to say that I had changed my mind and I really needed somewhere I could be looked after.

Along with the letter to Mr Priestman I also wrote one to Miss Beevers to tell her of my decision. I was going to pop it in her letterbox the next morning on my way to the university. But she saw me come to the gate and opened the front door.

'Oh, how nice to see you again,' she said. 'Come in and have another look round.'

She was so welcoming I didn't have the heart to tell her straightaway that I had changed my mind. So I went in and looked round the flat for the second time.

'Do you have a bicycle?' she asked.

'No.'

'Well, I have a bicycle I shall have to leave behind. Would you like to buy it?'

'Er – yes,' I said. 'How much do you want for it?'

'Just a pound would do. You know,' she went on, 'it's a real answer to prayer, your coming here.'

'Is it,' I said. 'Why?'

'Well, Mr Priestman has bought all my furniture and the money has been a great help towards my fare to India.'

I was beginning to wonder if I could ever tell her that I did not want her flat.

'Could you do something else for me?' she said.

'What's that?'

'I have a girls' class every Monday night. They're between fourteen and sixteen years old. They come and make things for missionaries and then we have a kind of epilogue, a blessing at the end of the evening. I wonder if you'd take that over for me.'

'Well,' I said, 'I don't know if I could manage it with everything else I have on.'

'Oh, don't worry,' she assured me. 'There are two other helpers who do it with me. They'll help you out. One is Winnie Griffin and the other is Nora Lazenby.'

She showed me where everything was kept.

'I'm sure you will enjoy it,' she said. 'It would be a real answer to prayer if you could take over. And there's a gentleman upstairs who is quite helpful.'

So that was that. I gave her the pound for the bicycle there and then. I thought it would save me some money in travelling expenses. As a matter of fact, that bicycle lasted me for years.

When I got to the university that day, I tore up the letters I'd written to Mr Priestman and Miss Beevers. I just couldn't face turning down the flat now.

The following Sunday I invited Miss Beevers to lunch at the Dorchester. She asked if she could bring a friend, and of course I said yes. It was the gentleman from the upstairs flat. He was handsome, and a little shy. He had a small neat moustache, which was fashionable at the time, and his short dark hair was greying at the temples. His name was Douglas Banks.

He did not say much during the meal. Miss Beevers – or Marjorie as I was soon used to calling her – did most of the talking. She was full of the mission she was to join and her preparations and hopes for her life in India. When we had finished lunch she had to be off somewhere. As she was going she put her hand on us both and said, 'Now look after each other while I'm away, won't you?'

Two weeks later Marjorie was about to set off and I was to take over the flat. She had a valedictory party and it was there that I met Douglas Banks again. Many of her friends were there from Trafalgar Street Church, the Evangelical Free Church of which Mr Priestman was an active member. Ken and Grace Gibbs ran a furniture store in the city. I met them for the first time at that party and they have remained life-long friends. Neville and Betty Collier were also there. Neville was a rather well-to-do solicitor, the church secretary at Trafalgar Street and well in with Mr Priestman.

Marjorie had asked Douglas Banks to show some films. He had an 8mm projector and collection of Charlie Chaplin films and the like.

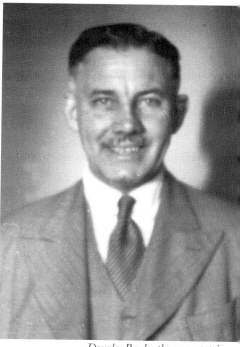

Douglas Banks, the man upstairs

He had a strong interest in amateur film-making and was one of the founder-members of the Cine Club in Hull. He was often asked to show his films by way of entertainment. To have a cine camera was quite a novelty at the time.

I remember thinking Douglas rather attractive. To tell the truth, whenever I was near him I felt aroused. He was quiet and seemed kind and gentle, and quite distinguished-looking. He didn't say much to me, in fact he hardly seemed to notice me, but while he was showing the films, I happened to be sitting near the projector and he put his hand on my shoulder. I felt a tremor go through me, and I kept thinking, oh dear, once again I'm getting attracted to somebody who isn't interested in me – for Douglas had never been other than rather cool and distant. It seemed to me that I was repeating the painful experience I had had with Douglas Johnson. He had let me down. Now here I was going through the same thing with another Douglas.

As soon as Marjorie had left for India, I moved into her flat. Because I now had somewhere of my own to live I invited the other girls on my course to come and have a flat-warming party. We had made a group booking for the ballet at the New Theatre. There was one ticket to spare. One of my group was an Indian lady called Mrs Darra and she said, 'Why not invite the man upstairs?'

'Oh, no,' I said, 'I don't know him.'

But she popped up and knocked on the door and asked if he'd come because we were one person short. He came down and we all went to the ballet, which we thoroughly enjoyed. After the show they all came back and had coffee with me, including Douglas.

Though we lived in the same house and I would hear him coming and going, we never saw much of each other. In fact we hardly spoke for weeks on end. He had the habit in the evenings of removing the jacket of his suit and putting on a silk dressing gown. Sometimes I'd see him going up the stairs in it. The material was in a tartan pattern. I remember thinking he looked so handsome in it. But he kept his distance.

I used to pay my rent through an estate agents called Holiday's. I knew that Douglas worked for Mr Holiday, so I wondered if I could pay it direct to him. It would save going all the way into town to do it. Catching him on the stairs one day I offered to hand the rent over to him.

'You don't pay me,' he said, rather brusquely it seemed to me. 'You have to pay it in to the office.'

He was so offhand it took me by surprise. He was almost discourteous, and I found him to be generally like that whenever I happened to meet him in the hall or on the stairs. He was certainly not friendly.

Still, it was my first term at the university. I had a lot of studying to do and I was meeting a lot of new people. I didn't have too much time to dwell on Douglas Banks' standoffish behaviour or to wonder seriously whether he was at all attracted to me.

As well as my student friends and tutors at the university, I got to know many people through Mr Priestman's church. I went regularly to the services. So did Douglas Banks. Along with Mr Priestman and several others, he had been founder-member of a Christian group which met in a room in Wright Street in the centre of Hull. As the group took on new members, larger premises were needed. Trafalgar Street Baptist was up for sale, so the group arranged the purchase and established their Evangelical Free Church.

Among the people to whom Mr Priestman introduced me were the Joelsons. They were a middle-aged Christian couple who were stalwart members of the church. Their hospitality to me was marvellous and it made me feel welcome in this strange new city.

One day, out of the blue, I got a letter from my brother Eddie to say he had just been stationed at Pocklington, a town not too far away. He had heard I was studying in Hull for a couple of years and he wanted to visit me in my new flat.

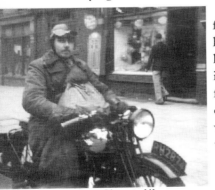

The day he arrived, there were workmen at the front of the house repairing bomb damage which had still not been seen to since the war. Because of his military background Eddie naturally took an interest in the work, and while I was making coffee for him in my flat, I heard him chatting away – to one of the workmen, I thought – outside my window. When he came in he said, 'I've just met that fellow who lives upstairs. Nice chap.'

'I don't know him,' I said.

'But he only lives upstairs.'

The man upstairs on his motorbike

'Oh, yes, I know,' I said. 'But I never see him.'

'Well, you ought to get to know him,' Eddie persisted. 'Tell you what, next time I see him I'll ask him where there's a good place to take you for dinner. It'll have to be earlyish though. I've got to catch the nine o'clock train tonight.'

Later that morning we went into town and had lunch at a nice little café called Jacksons. Then we had a good look round the centre of Hull. I was still getting to know the place myself, so it was an adventure for both of us. It was so good to be with Eddie again. He had been stationed in India for a long time, and also Ethiopia. I hadn't seen him for twelve years – since before the war in fact. We had such a lot to catch up on, and we ended the perfect day perfectly, with a lovely dinner at one of the places the man upstairs had suggested.

A week or so later Eddie booked me in for a long weekend at a hotel in Pocklington called The Three Feathers. He was looking for a flat for himself and his family, and had found one in York. We went to see it.

On the Saturday night he had arranged a big social event: a dance and cabaret. When he called for me, he was beautifully turned out in dress uniform. The next morning he escorted me to the local church. He was now a mature man of forty-five, so different from that gangling fourteen-year-old who had run away to the army all those years ago. He was splendid. I was so proud of him.

When we started at the university all the new students had to have a medical. Dr Rains, who examined me, told me I would have to have an X-ray.

When the results came back he asked to see me again. It seemed that there was a patch on my lung which he didn't like the look of. He questioned me about my family and their medical history as far as I knew it, and then made out an appointment card and told me to turn up at a certain address for further investigation. I found to my horror that it was a TB clinic.

They gave me a carton into which they wanted me to deposit some sputum. I didn't have much sputum, but they said I must try to bring up something. They feared I might have tuberculosis.

As soon as I got back to my flat I rang Auntie and told her they thought I had TB. Her response was immediate. 'Are you coming home for Christmas, dear?'

'Yes,' I said.

'Well, I'm taking you to Sweden. It might do you good.'

Fortunately, when the results came back it turned out not to be TB. But Auntie suggested we go to Sweden anyway. So that Christmas we flew to Stockholm. It was the first time I had ever been in an aeroplane.

Because flying was still something of a novelty, passengers were handed postcards of the plane, giving details of the speed and height of our flight. It occurred to me to send one to Douglas Banks. Auntie saw me writing. 'Who's that to?' she asked.

'The man upstairs,' I said, and told her a bit about him.

It was an amazing experience to be flying. Everything was so surprising. From the window of the plane, the islands below looked just like jewels in the sea.

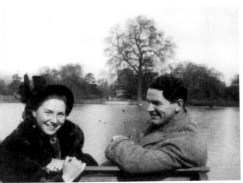

Newly-weds, Mabret and Gunnar

A few years earlier Auntie had gone to Sweden in search of her sister, with whom she had lost touch. It took weeks of following up one clue after another, arriving at one town only to be told that she had moved on, before the sister was eventually tracked down. With the sister was a little girl called Mabret who, during the war, had been found abandoned in a ditch, covered in sores and presumed orphaned. The sister had unofficially adopted Mabret, rather in the way that Auntie had adopted me.

Auntie's sister had since died, but for this trip we had been invited to stay with Mabret. Now in her twenties, a ravishing Swedish beauty, she was newly married to a fine-looking man called Gunnar. We landed at Gothenburg and drove through the city to where they had set up home.

The journey was beautifully picturesque. In every house a candle burned in the window, and in many of them hung a yellow and orange paper star, illuminated from within. It was the tradition in Sweden to light Santa Claus on his way. Even the trees lining the streets were lit up with fairy lights.

It was fascinating to celebrate Christmas with Mabret in the Swedish way. Instead of waiting until Christmas morning to open the presents, the whole family gathered around the Christmas tree on Christmas Eve and danced round it holding hands and singing carols. It was then that the giving and receiving of gifts took place. Instead of a turkey there was a traditional dinner of ling, a fish which had been prepared over the preceding eight or nine weeks. Much work goes into the preparation, but I'm afraid to say I didn't much care for the ling – nor did Auntie. It was rather pungent.

Instead of Christmas pudding they had a thick slab of pancakes piled high. It was cut into slices, much like a cake, and served with cream. That was much more to my taste. Delicious!

But by Christmas Day we were longing for more traditional fare. Auntie said, 'We'll have our own Christmas dinner, Mina. We'll go to a restaurant.'

None were open. Auntie would not be put off. We drove round and round until eventually we discovered a place used by lorry drivers where we could have the kind of Christmas dinner we were used to having at home. During our meal Auntie smiled at me and said, 'One day, child, your boat will come in.' She had said the same thing on other occasions. I just smiled back at her. My dear Auntie.

I arrived back in Hull on New Year's Eve. It had not seemed cold in Sweden because it was crisp and dry and all the buildings were centrally heated. Hull by comparison seemed much colder. Grey, damp and grisly.

As my train pulled in to Paragon station, Mr Joelson was waiting for me at the barrier. I was surprised to see him because I hadn't let anyone know when exactly I was getting back.

'How did you know I was coming on this train?' I asked him.

'I worked it out,' he said. 'I thought it would be this one. I'm taking you back to stay with us.'

'I should get back to Number Five. I have to start at the university again on Monday.'

'You're not going back to an empty house,' he said. 'Douglas isn't there. I've been trying to get in touch with him, but I think he must be with his relatives in Cleethorpes. He usually is, over the holidays. So Mother says you're to come home.' ('Mother' was what he called his wife.) 'She's got the room all ready for you. You're not spending New Year's Eve on your own in that empty house.'

So he took me to their home, and Mrs Joelson brought out some raisin wine. I felt very much at home. That evening was when I really got to know them. After that they were almost like family.

Their daughter Ruth was in her early twenties and training to be a doctor. She was a student at the Edinburgh Medical Mission and had invited a Norwegian student to stay over Christmas. The Joelsons had an ever-open door.

I had believed Ruth to be their only child, but that New Year's Eve they told me about their son, Bertie. They had never mentioned him before. He had run away from home, they said, when he was just a lad.

Later, when Ruth and I were alone together, she told me that Bertie had run off because he and his father did not get on. Mr Joelson was a strong Christian, with firm views. Bertie had become sick of it all and just wanted to get away. Up to that time they had not heard from him. When they did eventually get news that he was alive and well – many years later – it turned out that he had been abroad and bought land and had set himself up very nicely. I even put him up once, along with his wife and his two children, when he came back to see his parents again.

But all that was in the future. On this particular night we were seeing out the old decade, and seeing in the new one, and I must say the Joelson family were the best company to be in to do it. We looked forward to the Fifties. We had great hopes for the next decade as we moved away from the war years and into a time that surely promised peace and prosperity.

On New Year's day I felt I really had to get back to Eldon Grove. I had teaching practice at the Technical College and at the Western General Hospital for the following day and I needed to prepare for it. The Joelsons, of course, tried to persuade me to stay, but I insisted and prepared to return to an empty house.

When I got to the front door of Number Five, I saw there was a bag of groceries leaning against it, with the name 'Douglas Banks' on the label. I took it in with me to keep until he returned from Cleethorpes.

I had not been in long when I heard movement upstairs. I went up, groceries in hand, and knocked on the door of Douglas Banks' flat. There was no answer. I was just about to leave the groceries on the mat when the door opened, but by no more than an inch. From what I could see of him, Douglas Banks looked terrible. His eyes were sunken. He was unshaven.

'What's the matter with you?' I asked, really quite alarmed at his appearance.

'I've been ill,' he said, as brusquely as usual.

'This was left at the front door for you,' I said, handing him the bag of groceries.

'Yes, it's from the Arnolds,' he said as he grabbed for it. He later told me that the Arnolds were friends of his who also went to Trafalgar Street Church and often dropped round odd bits of shopping. At the time he said not much more than a muttered thank-you and closed the door again.

But he did look ill. I had been preparing a meal for myself, so I took up some soup and some lemon juice on a tray and banged on his door again. Again, it opened no more than an inch.

'Come on, don't be so foolish,' I said. 'I'm a nurse. Let me in.'

Grudgingly, he opened the door wider and I walked in.

'You get yourself on your bed,' I said. 'I've got this food for you. You've got to eat it.'

He didn't say much but I knew he was annoyed at the intrusion. I told him that the Joelsons had wondered what had happened to him.

'Have you been here all over the New Year?' I asked.

'Yes,' he said.

'The Joelsons thought you were away.'

He told me that he had been away over Christmas – with the Jacksons, who were his relatives in Cleethorpes. When he got back home he felt ill and so had just stayed in his room. It looked as though he had not eaten much more than bread and Lyons Golden Syrup. In fact, Lyons Golden Syrup seemed to be his staple diet. There were empty tins of it stacked around the kitchen.

He really did look awful. He hadn't shaved for days. He had great shadows under his eyes, and his stubble was becoming an untidy beard. It made him look like a down-and-out. He seemed sorry for himself and said less than he normally did. So after staying a few minutes longer to make sure that he was not seriously ill, I left him with the bit of food I had brought up and went back to my studies. It was a couple of weeks before I so much as saw him again.

Every Saturday night the Joelsons had a missionary meeting for China in their home and they had invited me to go along whenever I wished. One January evening I was just about to set out when I met Douglas Banks in the hallway. He asked where I was going and I said, 'The Joelsons.'

'I've got an appointment that way,' he said. 'Shall we get the bus together?'

'Are you coming to the meeting then?' I said, mildly surprised that he should be so forthcoming since he normally kept so much to himself.

'No. I've got to show some films.'

As we went on our way he explained that he was going to a YWCA meeting close to where the Joelsons lived. He was going to show his cine films. When we got off the bus – it was a tuppenny ride – he walked me to where the Joelsons lived and went on his way to the YWCA meeting. Mr Joelson let me in and introduced me to everybody – there were about eight people there, including Mrs Joelson. We had just begun when the bell rang. Mr Joelson opened the door and in walked Douglas Banks.

'What's happened?' I asked him.

'I made a mistake,' he said. 'It's the wrong date. It's next week, not this.'

'Well, Douggie,' said Mr Joelson, 'you might as well stay.'

And that's what he did, taking part in the meeting, and even leading the prayer at the close. When it was time to go, Douglas Banks offered to see me home – which was perfectly natural as he only lived upstairs. But I saw Mr and Mrs Joelson exchange knowing glances. I thought, 'If they only knew...'

Before we set off, Mrs Joelson invited me to pop in for Sunday afternoon tea the next day, and indeed any Sunday afternoon that I was at a loose end. She added that if anybody in my university study group had nowhere to go on a Sunday I was to bring them along too.

In fact, there was one girl in the group who was feeling quite miserable at the time and was not at all well. We called her Bunty. So the next afternoon I went again to the Joelsons and brought her along.

The Joelsons had an upright piano in the corner of their living room. At the sight of it Bunty at once brightened up and ran her hands over its shiny wood.

'What a beautiful piano,' she said. 'Very good condition.'

'Do you play?' asked Mrs Joelson.

'Yes, I do,' said Bunty.

'Well, go on, have a tinkle.'

She sat down and played beautifully. She was clearly an accomplished pianist. We seated ourselves round the table for tea, complimenting her on her obvious musical gift. At that moment the phone rang. Mr Joelson picked it up.

'Yes,' he said. 'Yes, she's here.' He looked across at me, and then at his wife, and put his hand over the receiver. 'There's something going on here,' he said to her with a twinkle in his eye. 'It's Douglas Banks again. Shall we invite him back after church?'

'Yes,' she said, 'Get him to come and have a bite with us.'

Mr Joelson turned back to the phone.

'Yes, we're all coming to church. You'd better come back with us and havesomething to eat.' So after tea we all went off to church and Douglas came back with us that evening.

We were having a few sandwiches and a drink when Mrs Joelson said to Bunty, 'Give us another tune, Bunty.' She played the Moonlight Sonata.

When we left the Joelsons, Douglas and I caught the bus and Bunty came with us. She was getting off at Cottingham Road to catch another bus to her digs when Douglas suggested we get off too and walk the rest of the way home. I thought it was a rather nice idea.

We waited at the bus stop with Bunty until her bus came along, and then Douglas took my arm – I was rather surprised at this new friendliness, but pleasantly so – and we started walking to Eldon Grove.

It was a clear cold evening. We arrived at Number Five and stood in the porch as Douglas got out his latchkey. It was then that he gave me a kiss. His cheek brushed against mine. I could feel the slight stubble.

'Your face is beautifully cool,' he said. His voice was low and gentle. There was something in its timbre which thrilled me to hear it. But the next thing he said was quite unexpected. 'You know, I'd love to give you a ring.'

I wondered what kind of ring he was talking about. Did he mean he wished to continue our conversation on the phone? Or could it be – surely not – his way of proposing to me?

I hardly saw anything of Douglas for the next week or so. It was as if nothing had happened. He even seemed to be avoiding me, or was that my imagination? I was so sad. I had thought for one moment that he felt something for me. And in that moment I had realised I felt something for him.

As the days passed I still didn't see much of him. I could sometimes hear him moving about in his flat upstairs. The living room was directly above mine. He was always in and out of the house, running up and down the stairs. Whenever we met by chance in the hall he never had much to say.

Then one day he came down and told me he had a meal ready, would I like to join him. I had been invited to have tea with one of the students on the course, a nice fellow called Stennet. It was to be at his lodgings. But it was such a surprise to be asked upstairs I forgot all about it. Douglas had that sort of effect on me. In any case I needed to know where I stood with him.

He had a large round pressure cooker – it looked like a bomb – and he prepared whole meals inside it. As we ate we began to talk about this and that. Near the end of the meal he said, 'I meant what I said, you know. I'm drawn to you. I want to give you a ring.'

'Do you?' I said. 'But you never speak to me.'

'No, well, this is all new to me,' he said. 'I've never been attracted to anyone in quite this way before.'

He had once been Secretary of the Young People's Fellowship at Trafalgar Street. I learned later that he used to invite them back to his flat and give them toast and tea after the evening service. Gradually they all got paired off, but he kept himself free. Several of them would have liked to get to know him better, but it was not until I came along, it seemed, that he became more interested. I told him about Douglas Johnson. He was saddened to hear my story, especially when I pointed out why his apparent indifference had so disturbed me. I felt the pattern was repeating itself. Was I starting to get involved with another Douglas only to discover that he was no more interested than the first?

He told me then that he was deeply attracted to me. He wept a little and told me about his parents who had died when he was only sixteen. I told him that I had lost my parents when I was even younger. We began to discover that we had a lot in common. For one thing, I found he was acquainted with a lot of the people I had met through Auntie – because they had come to Trafalgar Street and were connected with Mr Priestman.

There were other coincidences. He told me where he was born and I realised it was in the street right next to the one where I lived as a young girl in Leytonstone.

His father at that time had been quite prosperous. He owned a yacht and a large chauffeur-driven car, which in 1910 was something rather special. We laughed at the similarity of our parents' Christian names. His father was called Edward Albert, mine Albert Edward. His mother was Anna-Marie, mine Hannah Matilda – and both had given birth to us when they were in their early forties.

What he told me about Mr Holiday explained a lot. I had not liked the look of Mr Holiday on the few occasions I had seen him when paying in my rent. What I heard now confirmed my view. When he had heard a nurse was coming to take the flat, he had teased Douglas. 'That'll be a nice young lady for you, then,' he had said.

Douglas had replied that he would have nothing to do with me. And for a long time, of course, he certainly didn't have anything to do with me. The reason he felt so strongly about it, he said, was that he had been at Marjorie's beck and call. Whenever there was a tap dripping or a fuse to be mended, she used to run to him for

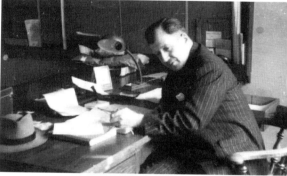
Mr Cyril Holiday

help. The whole house had suffered minor bomb damage during the war and he had taken on the responsibility of gradually making repairs to the place for Mr Priestman. He was frankly getting fed up with it all. What Mr Holiday had said was the last straw. He thought he had enough to see to – without getting involved with yet another tenant in the house.

The talk we had together that evening made me feel much closer to Douglas. Funnily enough, he still would not take my rent. I had to continue paying it in to the Holiday office in Scale Lane. He did not like to mix his business and private life, and he was probably quite right in that. He had the utmost integrity. It was one of the many things I admired in him.

Finally, we got down to the practical side of things. We set a date for our engagement. It was to be the seventh of March and we would have a party and invite all our friends to celebrate.

I did not write much in my diary around that time, except for the occasional appointment for my work, but that night I wrote one simple sentence:

Friendship is a wonderful thing.

The next day I had to give a lecture at the technical college. It was actually about the composition of the air around us, and how important it is for our health. I opened the lecture with the words 'I'm walking on air' because that's the way I felt. It seemed an appropriate way to start.

After the lecture I went on to the university. When the girls saw me they said, 'Where have you been?'

'Why?' I asked.

'Well, Dr Stern has been looking for you. You had an appointment with him this morning. Don't you remember? He wanted to go over your papers with you.'

Dr Alex Stern was our psychology tutor. I had forgotten all about the appointment, which I was meant to fit in before my lecture. Before I went to see him and apologise, I thought I had better explain to the girls why I was not altogether myself.

'As a matter of fact,' I said, 'I *am* walking on air. I had a proposal of marriage last night.'

There was much excitement and congratulations. Then we remembered my appointment with Dr Stern. 'You're supposed to report to him straightaway,' they said.

When I finally got to see Dr Stern he asked why I had not turned up for our meeting. His brows were furrowed and his expression was living up to his name. I decided to tell him the absolute truth. I explained that I had had a proposal the night before and it had put the appointment entirely out of my mind. To my surprise, his attitude changed immediately.

'Oh, in that case,' he said with a broad smile, 'I forgive you. And congratulate you. You know, you'll be all the better for this as a tutor. You'll understand better how others feel. I know that sounds strange, but you will.'

We went through my papers and case histories. They were not good, but he was understanding about it all and before I left he congratulated me again and wished me all the best.

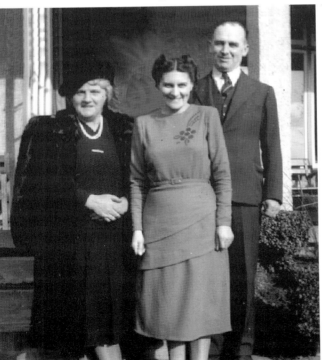

Not long afterwards I bumped into Mr Stennet. 'What happened to you yesterday?' he enquired. 'I looked out for you but you didn't come to tea.'

'No, I didn't,' I said. 'I'm afraid I was just too busy.'

As soon as I could, I rang to tell Auntie that someone had proposed to me.

'Who it is, dear?' she asked, a little apprehensively.

'The man upstairs,' I said.

She was not happy.

With Auntie and, behind me, Bob Hutchinson inching his way in

11

Not Somehow…

Can the wedding guests fast while the bridegroom is with them?
Mark 2.19

On Monday the seventh of March, 1950, Douglas made this entry in his diary:

> Very busy day. First of month collection. Back at 4.30. Called at shop re
> cheese not sent. Did my books then helped Mina to clean the Covenantor
> Room for tomorrow evening. Worked till 1 am. Room looks wonderful.

We were preparing for our engagement party. The Covenantor Room was a
large area above my flat at the back of the house. It was used every Sunday
afternoon for meetings of the Covenantors who were a group of young Christian
men and boys, mainly from Trafalgar Street Church. They came for Bible study
with Mr Priestman, who had started the group. As with the rest of Number
Five, Douglas looked after the room, got it ready for the meetings, and could use
it whenever he wanted. At one end was a small kitchen and a gas fire. After their
meeting the Covenantors would sit round sipping tea and eating crumpets,
toasted by the fire and spread with various potted pastes. At the other end was a
full-size billiard board. When its wooden covers were in place, it made an ideal
table for serving the food at parties.

In the next day's entry Douglas wrote:

> Up at 6.30. Breakfast 7.30. Collecting till 4.30. To Lee's to collect ring. To
> Medley's for 1 doz bread rolls. 6/-. 2 bottles of squash. Balanced my books
> and 7 o'clock to Covenantor Room for the engagement celebration. About 36
> people present. Mostly Mina's student friends.

All my student friends came. One of them had a Christmas cake left over
and she brought that. Dr John Bradley, our chemistry tutor, brought his violin
and played it. Some of Douglas's friends were there too, of course. Miss Olive
Priestman was there to represent the Priestman family and Mr Joelson made an
excellent Master of Ceremonies. Arthur Coultas, a great friend of Douglas, lived
in the Avenues the other side of Pearson Park in a beautifully converted attic
flat. It would be called a penthouse now. Arthur was a cultured man with an

extensive collection of classical music on 78 rpm records. In particular he loved the works of Richard Wagner. He now proposed a toast to Douglas.

As the evening wore on, Mrs Joelson became increasingly upset. Douglas had still not produced the ring. When it looked as though the party was coming to an end she came over to me. 'Have you got it yet?' she asked. She was angry by this time.

'No,' I said, slightly anxious myself that Douglas had changed his mind about the whole thing.

'I'm going to have a word with him,' she said.

'No, don't, please.' I didn't want a fuss made. It would be too embarrassing.

Ten minutes later, Douglas stopped me at the top of the stairs outside his flat. There was nobody else around. He pulled out the ring and pushed it on to my finger. It slid on beautifully.

When I got back to the room I was desperately trying to show the ring off. Nobody noticed at first. Eventually Mrs Joelson looked down at my finger and said, 'My goodness, at last.' She was always outspoken.

That weekend I visited Cleethorpes for the first time to meet Douglas's relatives. I was scared stiff. His Uncle Charlie had been a painter and decorator and now owned a small shop. His wife Bertha was by that time an invalid. Cousins Doris and Bertie Jackson were the people Douglas had been staying with at Christmas.

Cleethorpes was a small seaside town which attracted holidaymakers in the summer. It had a long stretch of amusement arcades along the promenade, and a small fairground. To get there meant taking the ferry across the Humber to a place called New Holland and then catching the train to Cleethorpes. It took about an hour-and-a-half.

The train came in along the sea front. The holiday season had not yet begun. The fairground was closed up and deserted. The tide was out. There was no sea to be seen, only muddy sand stretching to the horizon. We arrived at the station at around eleven o'clock and made our way to the shop. As we entered I could see Bertha lying on the bed in the room just behind the shop. I almost lost my nerve, but Douglas said, 'Just be your natural self. You'll be fine.'

Of course he was right. Charlie welcomed us in, sat us down and brought in a tray of tea. In no time we were chatting away to him and his wife as if I had known them for years.

For lunch Douglas and I went round the corner to the Cosy Café, then had a walk along the promenade before catching the train back to Hull. On a later weekend we stayed overnight at the Jacksons and got to know them. I shared a room with Doris's mother, Grace Schofield. She told me all about Douglas's parents. She said, 'Oh, Mina, they would have loved you. His mother was lovely and she would have been so happy for you.'

The following weekend it was Douglas's turn to meet Auntie Dagmar. Mabret was visiting with her husband Gunnar. On Friday the seventeenth of March Douglas wrote:

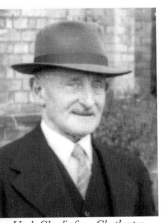

Uncle Charlie from Cleethorpes

Up at 6.30. CB [cold bath] and breakfast. 8 o'clock to office. 11 am to station for 12.20 to Kings Cross. Mina was 20 mins late. Began to think she would miss the train! Got good seat. Nice bright day. Took snack in train. Arrived K.Cross 5.25. Was met by Gunnar and Mabret. By 73 bus to Sheen Court and walked up Sheen Common Drive to Cornerways [Auntie's house]. Had a wonderful meal after meeting Auntie and May.

SATURDAY 18 MARCH: Slept in a lovely south side room which I am told was given up to me by Auntie. Mina brought me tea and biscuits at 7.30. Up at 8 o'clock. CB. Down to breakfast 8.45. Missed Gunnar and Mabret. 10 am morning prayers and out to Kew Gardens in the Ford [Auntie's car]. Nice sunny day. Took some cine pictures in Kew. Back to dinner [this is what he called lunch] at 12.30. About 16 people there!

Auntie loved having a lot of people around her and was always inviting them to her house. Though he put a good face on it, Douglas was not good at meeting new people. He was a little shy and it upset him rather. His diary continues:

Into lounge to see some cine pictures. Tea 6 o'clock. Harold Brocklebank arrived on bus at 7. Saw some more pictures and had supper 9.30.

Harold was an old friend of Douglas. They had met at art class in the early twenties. Harold now lived in London. He was to be best man at our wedding.

SUNDAY 19 MARCH: Up at 7.30 after a cup of tea brought in by Mina! CB and down to breakfast with Gunnar and Mabret. Very sunny. Took some cine pictures of breakfast table. 10.45 to Duke Street Church. Alan Redpath [one of our mutual acquaintances] not there. Place taken by Rev Keith Samon. 1.30 dinner [lunch] and stayed in writing and getting some things from the attic. [Auntie turned out curtains and so on – for us to take back with us.] 5 o'clock tea and cakes and a rush in the car to Buckingham Palace and round the Mall to Portman Street Baptist Church. 8.10 Frantic dash to Kings Cross. Arrived 9.10. Left 9.20. In Hull 2.30 am. Got a taxi to No. 5. 3/6. Quickly got to bed. Up at 7.30 to office to do rate notices till 5.30.

Douglas worked so hard for Mr Holiday but earned so little it is amazing he could afford a taxi for us. We seldom used one after that. From time to time Mr Holiday would give Douglas chickens, or packets of sugar, to supplement his income. I didn't like it. I once went to the office and told Mr Holiday what I thought of him. 'If you paid Douglas a decent wage,' I said, 'we could buy these things ourselves.'

At Kew Gardens

He was earning £5 a week at the time. He never earned any more to the day he retired. It was a job of real dedication, and Douglas had such integrity about it. If he had books to balance, or other outstanding office work to do, he would keep at it until after midnight even though he received nothing in the way of overtime or bonus payments. He had worked for Holiday's since before the war. Mr Holiday had kept the job open for Douglas when he was called up and Douglas was grateful to be able to return to it. Mr Holiday was a good deal older than Douglas. There was some sort of understanding, a gentlemen's agreement, that Douglas would take over the business himself when Mr Holiday retired. That was the promise that kept Douglas going, and gave him such commitment to the firm. He was to work for Mr Holiday for the next fifteen years.

Auntie was a woman who was easily flattered by the attentions of men. She was used to it, and those who brought her flowers and said the things she liked to hear found it easy to get round her and win her approval. In this manner, I am sorry to say, she was taken in by several who were interested only in her wealth and influence. Douglas was not that kind of man at all. He was always down to earth and real. He would not say anything to anybody which he did not believe. He certainly was not the kind to play up to Auntie in the way she was used to. As a result they did not really hit it off. She considered him not good enough for me. Admittedly, things were going to be difficult for us at first since we had so little money, but I knew in my heart that Douglas was right for me and that somehow we would get through. But Auntie was the nearest I had to a mother and knowing what she thought made me deeply upset.

On a cold day at the end of April it snowed. Douglas was suffering from lumbago. It did not help that he had to be out on his bike in all weathers, collecting the rents. We had received a letter from Auntie that day containing a one pound note. We decided to go to the university film society to see a double bill, *The Strange Cabinet of Dr Caligari* and *Brief Encounter*. It was the latter film that stayed in my mind.

We were still living separately, each in our own flat. But preparations had to be made for the time, following the wedding and honeymoon, when we would both move into Douglas's flat. Early in May we started sorting through his attic rooms at the top of the house.

Douglas was not good at throwing things away and there was an awful jumble of all sorts of old electrical and photographic oddments which we tried to clear out. Much of it just got transferred from the large attic room to a small room at the back.

Douglas was also working on the kitchen, which was in a poor state. New wood was still rationed: one needed coupons for it. But Douglas managed to get some old painted wood, second hand. He had to strip down every bit to the original surface before it could be used. But he was clever at woodworking and furnished the whole kitchen with fitted cupboards, each individually carpented.

Douglas's health was not improving. His lumbago was getting worse and he was also complaining of stomach pains. At the end of May he had a thorough examination, blood tests and an X-ray at the Western General Hospital. A couple of days later he was given a barium meal. According to the examining doctor, the results showed that there was absolutely nothing wrong with him physically. He put down the symptoms to nerves. Perhaps, I thought, he was getting worried about marrying me!

Our first weekend away alone together was at Scarborough. Douglas managed to get the Friday off. It was the twenty-third of June – his birthday:

> Nice warm day. Caught the 9.25 bus to Scarborough. Arrived 12 o'clock. Down into Italian Gardens for our sandwiches and some snaps. To the Chessington Guest House. Fixed up for the weekend, B&B. Then went round shops. Dinner at the Georgian 7/- at 5.30. To Northend for Fol De Rols at 7 o'clock. No queue. 2/6 each. Not too good. Walked back 10 o'clock. Bed 11 o'clock.

> SATURDAY 24 JUNE: Up 7 am. Breakfast 8 am. Caught 9.15 bus to Ravenscar. Met Arthur Coultas. Showed us a deserted village. Walked along cliff tops to Robin Hood's Bay. Had some dinner on the cliffs from the fish and chip shop. Got our feet wet when a wave rushed up at the causeway. Walked back along the beach, Mina paddling, to Ravenscar. Tea at a café and caught the 4.20 bus back to Scarborough for 6 pm dinner at Chessington. To the Metro. Saw *The Young Musician.*

> SUNDAY 25 JUNE: Up 8 o'clock. V. good breakfast at 9 am. Cereal and bacon, sausages and egg. 10 am up Oliver's Mount. Took some photos. Came down at noon. Just got to Chessington in time for dinner at 1 pm, finishing up with ice cream and peaches. Caught the 2.20. Arrived Hull 5 o'clock. Something to eat. Trafalgar Street for evening service.

Towards the end of July preparations were reaching fever pitch. I was straightening up my flat downstairs prior to giving it up and was then going down to London to shop for my trousseau and stay at Auntie's until the wedding. Douglas finished off painting and papering the kitchen. The materials cost nine pounds nineteen shillings, which was quite a lot of money – twice Douglas's weekly wage. Builders and plumbers were forever in and out. Arthur Coultas helped us to lay two carpets and carry furniture up to the large attic room which we were making into an extra bedroom. My furniture arrived from London and there was a bedroom suite of two single beds and bedside tables which all had to be unpacked and arranged in place. That Saturday afternoon Douglas saw me off on the London train. I was to stay down there for the next month and would not see him again until the wedding.

I visited many of my old friends but I wrote to Douglas almost every day, wherever I was staying. He was still worrying while I was away, but he had a sense of humour about it, as this entry from his diary indicates:

WEDNESDAY 25 JULY: Up 6.15. Couldn't sleep after six o'clock, worrying about my book on How To Stop Worrying And Live Happily!

I had met up with an old friend, Vera Merry, one of the workers from the Lansdowne Place Medical Mission. We went into London to buy the materials for my trousseau. Then I went back to Auntie's, where I was staying.

Not long after I arrived Auntie told me she had received a letter from Eric Doyle. It was in reply to the wedding invitation: he could not come. I was sorry about that. We had been through so much together during the war, I would have liked him to have been there.

'You should have married him,' she said. 'You wouldn't have had all this worry.'

By 'worry' she meant what she saw as our poor financial state. I was stung by her refusal to understand what Douglas meant to me. He certainly meant more to me than material riches.

'If Eric wanted to marry me, why didn't he say anything to me?' I retorted. 'He never even mentioned the word love. Anyhow,' I went on, 'the Lord has brought us together. Douglas is a Christian and he's pure gold. The Lord has been saving us for each other. I'm convinced of it.'

I reminded Auntie of what she had said when I was so upset about Douglas Johnson: 'The Lord has something far better for you.' I pointed out the coincidence that I'd had two Douglases and two Erics in my life, and I quoted Mark 12.11: 'This is the Lord's doing. It is marvellous in our eyes.'

'Anyhow,' I concluded, 'I think I'll go back to Hull, to Douglas, and finish my preparations for the wedding there.'

That upset her. She realised she had hurt me. 'Why don't you go to the flat at Brighton?' she said to me more gently. 'Ask Mary to go with you.'

But I was not to be won round that easily. 'No, I won't ask Mary. I'll ask Margaret.'

Auntie had clung on to my sister Mary since I had brought her round one day and introduced her. She was entranced by her talent for running up dresses and making beautiful cakes and so on, and would get her to do all sorts of things for her. I did not want to give Auntie the satisfaction of getting everything her own way. It was a battle of wills, I suppose. I had chosen Douglas on my own and for myself and knew he was right for me. I wanted to continue to show my independence. Being in charge of my own trousseau was part of it.

Margaret was Mary's daughter. She was now twenty-one and had been married to Fred Samuels for four years. When she heard that I was getting married she sent a card to Douglas:

I hear you are hoping to marry my aunt. You better look after her. If not you'll have me to deal with!

She was to be my bridesmaid. We had a delightful week in Brighton together. We went out to fish and chip shops for our meals. Like her mother, she was good with her fingers and made up a dress for me and decorated a hat in preparation for another wedding that Auntie and I were shortly to attend.

We talked, of course, about marriage and having children. I told her about Mabret and Gunnar. They were wanting to start a family. Mabret was about Margaret's age, but at forty-one I was a late starter. I was still longing to have a child. I had always thought I'd like at least six. I imagined them all sitting round the table. Maybe that was expecting too much by now, but I would be happy to have just one child by Douglas. As it turned out, within the year all three of us – Margaret, Mabret and myself – were expecting our first child.

I returned to Hull towards the end of August. It seemed I had been away from Douglas for so long. We talked until midnight. I had moved out of my flat downstairs before I left for London. Clearly,

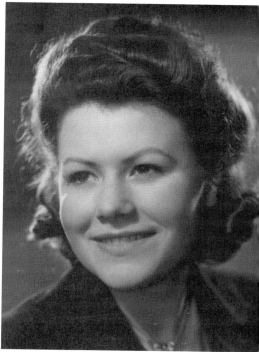

My niece Margaret Samuels, 1950

I could not stay with Douglas before the wedding – though it was only a few weeks away and I was longing to live with him – so I arranged with Mrs Tranmore, the next door neighbour, to stay those last weeks with her. But I must confess that at night Douglas would leave the front door off the latch and in the early hours I would creep out of Mrs Tranmore's house and up to Douglas and get into bed with him.

At the beginning of September I went back down to stay with Auntie again, this time until the wedding. Auntie was resigned to the wedding now. She was paying for the reception and had organised the whole thing. She upset Douglas by getting all the flowers. He wanted to arrange that. However, the bouquet she got me was undeniably beautiful, a mix of pink silk roses, love-in-a-mist and lily-of-the-valley. They remained through the years to remind us of our wedding day.

I was getting nervous as the day approached. All those usual anxieties. Was I doing the right thing? What if Auntie's misgivings proved correct? A couple of days before the big day, I went to Kings Cross to meet Douglas on his arrival. I saw a group of people, among whom I thought I spotted Douglas. But what was this? He seemed almost bald. I knew he had been worrying in the previous few months, but surely this wasn't the man I was about to marry?

Fortunately, it wasn't. It was somebody completely different. In my anxiety I had mistaken him for my Douglas. When I saw the handsome figure of Douglas approaching me with a wave and a smile, my heart flooded with joy. This was the man I was going to marry.

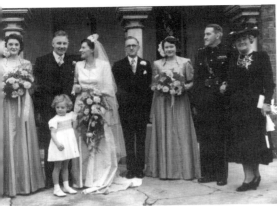

To my left, Harold Brocklebank, Margaret Samuels, Eddie, and Auntie, and to Douglas's right, Eddie's daughter, Peggy

The wedding ceremony was held on the sixteenth of September 1951 at a Baptist church in Gunnersbury. There was an inscription outside above the door: FOX'S MARTYRS. Unfortunately, one of the wedding photographs shows Douglas posed directly under the word 'Martyr'!

A reception followed at Chiswick Town Hall, just across the road from the church. There were around two hundred and fifty people invited. When it was over, Douglas and I went into a little room set aside for us to change into our travelling clothes. We were intending to leave directly for our honeymoon. Douglas had arranged it all. I knew it was somewhere abroad because he said I would need my passport. But he kept our destination firmly to himself. He wanted it to be a surprise.

We packed our wedding clothes into one case, which was to be left behind

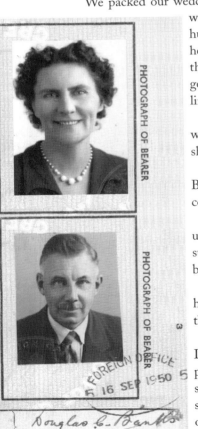

with Auntie. Our other case was for the trip. We were in a hurry to catch our train and after I had got my things on I helped Douglas get his things together. We came out into the hall in a big hurry. Everybody had lined up to say goodbye. I reached out my hand to the first person in the line – and found one of Douglas's socks on it!

We scrambled into the taxi. The driver asked where we were going. Auntie pushed a suitcase into the front and shouted, 'Victoria!'

Actually, we had first planned to have tea with Harold Brocklebank and his mother. 'No, not Victoria,' I quickly corrected. 'Morden!'

We set off, waving our goodbyes to the crowd behind us. We were well on our way when we discovered that the suitcase we had with us was the one which should have been left behind.

'We haven't got the right case!' I shouted to the driver. 'I haven't got my honeymoon clothes in here!' We had to go all the way back to pick up the right one.

It turned out that Douglas had booked a holiday in Dijon, in the south of France. But when we raced into the port, with only minutes to spare before the scheduled sailing time, we discovered that the weather was so bad no ship was making the crossing. The only ferry that was still operational was to the channel island of Jersey. The travel agents suggested that this would be the best place for our honeymoon. We seemed to have little choice.

When we arrived on board, the purser was about to put Douglas in a cabin with a crowd of others at one end of the ship, and me in a single cabin at the other end of the ship. I said, 'Look, we can't be separated like that. We've just got married.' Eventually, we were given a cabin together. It was near the boiler room and very noisy.

It was a terrible crossing. The ship was up and down, and so were we. We hadn't been in the cabin long when Douglas was hanging over the basin.

'What's the matter?' I asked him.

'I think I must go out on deck and get some fresh air. I don't feel too good.'

'You're not sea-sick, are you? You shouldn't be sea-sick with a skipper for a father.' I said. 'I'm never sea-sick. I came home from Malta in terrible weather and I wasn't sea-sick.'

But Douglas just had to go up on deck and walk around for a bit. He left me in the cabin. When he came back, he found me hanging over the basin.

When we arrived at last at St Helier there was a placard advertising Swansdown Hotel, the hotel we were booked into. I thought it sounded rather romantic and fit for a honeymoon. We climbed shakily into the courtesy bus and were dropped at the entrance to the hotel. Unsteadily, we walked up to the reception desk. I was just about to write 'Staerck' in the visitors' book, when Douglas nudged me and whispered, 'No, not that.'

The whole fortnight remained bitterly cold. I gingerly had a dip one day, and Douglas took a photograph. He couldn't bring himself even to paddle.

We had brought all the wedding cards and greetings telegrams with us. A card which had accompanied some flowers from the Zenana Bible and Medical Mission bore the words: NOT SOMEHOW BUT TRIUMPHANTLY. Immediately they struck us as rather appropriate. I put the card to one side and when we got home and were settling in, I wedged it in the frame of a wedding picture. There it remains to this day.

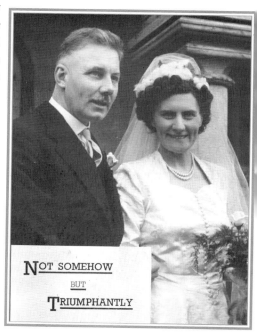

NOT SOMEHOW
BUT
TRIUMPHANTLY

12

A Son

For to us a child is born, to us a son is given
Isaiah 9.6

Around the Easter of 1951, Ethel Izzard came to stay with us for the weekend. I was sitting playing at the piano, when out of the blue she said, 'Mina, aren't you pregnant?'

I stopped and looked at her. 'No, of course not,' I replied, and went on with whatever it was I was playing.

'Well, I think you are,' she persisted. 'I can tell by your back.'

I dismissed the idea at first. But then, when I mentioned it to Douglas that evening, he pointed out that I taken quite a fancy to oranges. I had eaten twelve the previous evening.

I went along to see our GP, Dr Cummings. He took a sample of my urine and told me he would let me know the result. The pregnancy test used live mice in those days. A day or two later I visited him again.

'You're not pregnant,' he said. 'You've killed all the mice.' He was joking – I think. 'All the same,' he went on. 'I suppose we should do another test just to make sure.' This time the test proved positive. Ethel Izzard had been right.

Auntie Dagmar was in the habit of granting annuities to people in need. Missionaries all over the world were supported by her in this way. When she heard that I was pregnant she told me she was going to arrange an annuity for

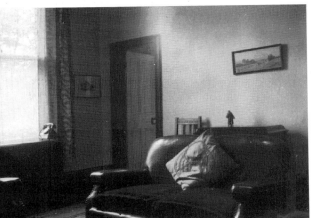

me, so there would be some money for the child. It would amount to £52 each year – a pound a week. She went on to tell me that her solicitor had recently received a request which he felt was worthy of her attention. A young boy had won a place at university but his father could not afford to keep him there.

'You know the father,' she said. 'It's Douglas Johnson.'

I was shocked.

The flat upstairs

'But you're not going to give him the money, are you?' I felt weak at the thought of it.

'Well,' she replied, 'it's not the son's fault, is it?'

Much as I understood her reasoning, I could not go along with it. It upset me that she would even consider it. It felt like a betrayal.

When Auntie finally came to visit us in Hull she took a dim view of Number Five. She was used to a high degree of luxury. The flat upstairs, where Douglas and I were now living together, must have seemed very shabby to her.

I was not happy with the state of the place, but we had made certain improvements. We intended to do more and I hoped eventually that we would move to something better. A house, or bungalow perhaps, on the outskirts of the city, away from the bombsites and the grimy streets and the smell of fish that characterised Hull in the Fifties. Auntie wanted us to move down to London. She even arranged the possibility of a good job for Douglas down there, but he refused to consider the idea.

She had brought me the material for a wicker cradle for the baby, and she was going to ask Mary to make it up for me. I said no. I wanted to do it myself.

Douglas was decorating the attic walls, papering them and painting the woodwork. I painted a seascape over the wallpaper and made a pretty cradle. It had little curtains and was padded inside. Auntie was quite taken with it. She asked if Mabret could have it when my baby had grown out of it. Mabret's baby was due a few months after mine.

I didn't want to get rid of the cradle because I was still hoping we would have more children after this first one. But because Mabret was much younger than me, I suppose Auntie felt there would be a greater likelihood of her going on to have other children.

By this time I had completed my sister tutor training course at the university. The practical part, the teaching practice at the Western General Hospital, I managed to fit it in before I became too pregnant. The theoretical part of my course at Hull University came to an end before the summer and culminated in an exam. Since it was an extramural course, I had to go to London for it. A few weeks later I heard that I had passed. My brother Eddie, now living in York with his family, was able to come across to Hull for the graduation ceremony.

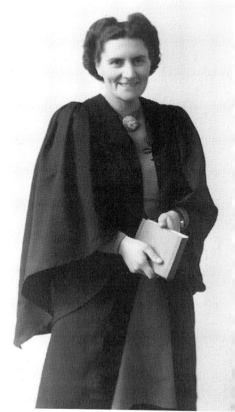

Graduation, 1951

* * *

One of the people we saw a lot of at the time was Stella Mathison. Douglas had known her since 1923. They were both the same age and had gone to the same church. Early on they had lived near one another. She had invited him to her twenty-first birthday party and a few months later he invited her to his.

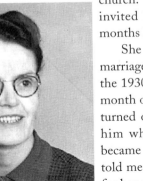
Stella Mathison

She had been married twice and had one son from each marriage. Her first husband had died of consumption during the 1930s when her son Charlie Tomson was no more than a month old. Some years later she married a Mr Mathison who turned out to be a terrible drinker. She was forced to leave him when her second son Malcolm was a toddler. She became depressed and was close to taking her own life. She told me that it was only because of Douglas, and his concern for her and the children, that she did not.

When Douglas had told her he was going to marry me, she was furious. It seemed she had hoped he would eventually marry her, though it was not something she had ever mentioned to Douglas. However, to her credit, she managed to reconcile herself to the fact that I was to be his wife, and she soon became a good family friend.

I had invited her to tea one day when I was preparing for the examination. For practice, I was dissecting hearts in the kitchen. I had a human heart, a sheep's heart and a frog's heart all laid out on the table when the bell rang. At the door was a boy who looked like a young Adonis. He wore a lovely white shirt and his hair was golden. It was Malcolm Mathison. He was about fourteen. He had come to tell me that Stella would be along soon. She was just doing some last-minute shopping.

'I've got to go back and meet her in ten minutes,' he said. 'Help carry the bags.'

I thought he would be quite interested in the dissection so I invited him in for a moment. 'Come along, I've something to show you,' I said.

We went upstairs and I showed him the dissected hearts. I practised my lecture on him, pointing to my anatomical chart and indicating where the heart was positioned in the body and how it functioned. He seemed interested enough and asked some intelligent questions before going off to meet his mother.

He told her I was looking forward to having them for tea. I had got everything prepared, he said, and he even knew what food they were going to be eating. Heart sandwiches!

The baby was due in September. I was booked into Townsend Nursing Home, a hospital for women on Cottingham Road. My obstetrician was a Dr Richard George Winchester. He looked after me throughout my pregnancy.

It was the day of Harvest Festival. We had several people to Sunday tea, including the Joelsons, and then we went on to the evening service at Trafalgar Street. Mrs Joelson was sitting next to me. I was in some discomfort. I whispered in her ear, 'When labour starts, do you get wind?'

'No,' she said, dismissively. 'You'll know when it starts all right.'

But I couldn't settle. Douglas was on my other side. I kept asking him the time.

'You know, every two minutes you ask me what time it is,' he said at last. 'Are you all right?'

'Yes,' I said. 'I've just got wind.'

After the sermon, I was still uncomfortable. Douglas suggested that we should get back home. I agreed. As we were leaving, Neville Collier offered us a lift. Thanks, we said, but the bus would be fine; it took us straight to our door.

We stood at the bus stop for some time. When the bus came it was full and passed without stopping. It was a fine evening, so we walked home instead.

As soon as we got home, I ran a bath and had a soak. I had packed a case all ready to go into the hospital. The only thing I had left to do was wash my hair. When I got back to the bedroom, I calmly folded a large white sheet and put it on the bed. 'What's that for?' asked Douglas.

'In case the waters break,' I replied.

'I'm going to ring them up,' he said, alarmed.

'Oh, don't ring them up. They'll think I'm making a fuss.'

But he was getting nervous. He rang Townsend and they told him to bring me in. 'Don't worry,' they assured him, 'If it's a false alarm she can come home again in the morning.' Douglas rang for a taxi. I got to the hospital just as labour began. It lasted almost ten hours. The baby's head appeared around ten o'clock the next morning. 'It's a boy,' said the midwife and she put him into my arms.

'Oh, my lovely David,' I said. 'Oh, David, you're beautiful.'

'Is that his name?' she asked.

'That's going to be his name. Yes,' I answered.

It was a Monday and Douglas was working. He had rung the hospital an hour earlier and was told there was no news. When he rang again at lunchtime he was told, 'You're the father of a son. They're both very well.' He finished work early and got to the hospital at around three in the afternoon. He brought a photograph with him of himself when he was two days old. When the nurses saw it they asked, 'Have the photographers been already?'

'No,' I said. 'My husband brought it. It's of him when he was just born. But doesn't it look like David?'

My first visitor after Douglas was Mrs Joelson. They asked her if she was a relative. She said, 'Yes. Sort of.'

'She's the only granny David will know,' I said to them.

She had a big bag with her. 'Do you know what I've got here?' she said. 'A meat pie and an apple tart for Douglas. I'm going along there now to see that he has them.'

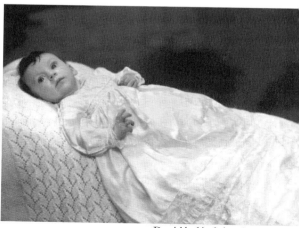

David in his christening gown

I remained in Townsend for another week. By the time I came home Douglas had made a corner of our bedroom into a nursery. On the walls he had painted fairies and cherub faces. David looked so much at home in his little cradle.

Since graduating, I had the qualifications to become a sister tutor, but I could not immediately go back to the Western General and start teaching full-time because there was David to look after. Douglas was still working hard for Mr Holiday, until midnight sometimes, balancing his books. So for that first year of David's life I was a housewife and mother. I enjoyed it very much.

Our first car was an Austin Seven. We called it Ruby. I don't remember why. Perhaps because the interior was red. The car itself was black. But it was a dear little thing. David was about five or six months old when we got it.

In the first year of our marriage and before, Douglas had driven me about the place on his large motorcycle. Even when I was quite heavily pregnant we would go on long trips into the country. Now that David was with us, we had to use public transport or carry him on our bicycles. Since we lived close to the centre of the city the bus service was quite good. At the top of Eldon Grove was the big main thoroughfare into town, Beverley Road, and it was well served by a wide variety of buses. At that time there were also electrically propelled trolley buses, powered by overhead cables.

My bicycle – the one I had bought for £1 from Marjorie Beevers – had a basket at the front and, dangerous though it might sound now, I just used to sit David in there whenever I had to take him anywhere. Douglas had a special little seat fixed to the back of his pushbike and we would often go out on little excursions, taking it in turns to carry David. There was not the volume of traffic that there is now, and many people used bicycles in Hull because most of the city is so flat. But Douglas had long wanted a car of his own.

At that time few people owned a car. But Douglas had a driving licence and had learned to drive years earlier – before it was necessary to take a test – and the day came when he felt it was time to find a little car for ourselves. And so, with our meagre savings, Ruby was bought and delivered to our front door.

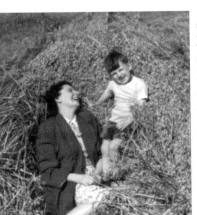

We decided to take our first trip in it to Hornsea, a seaside town about twenty miles away, where Stella Mathison had a flat. We got all packed up and into the car, ready for our excursion. Douglas was a little nervous. He had not driven a car since before the war. He slowly drove to the top of the Grove – all of one hundred yards – but when we reached Beverley Road he felt there was rather too much traffic, so we turned round and went back to the house again.

But he soon got used to driving again. Within a few weeks it was as if Ruby was part of the family.

I loved that little car. David did too. He would be asleep on my lap on our many trips out and I felt I could

Sunk Island, summer 1953

just relax and watch the countryside. There was a sun-roof, and large cloth pockets in the door where I could keep everything to hand. The dashboard was of rosewood, and the upholstery was a dark red leather which gave off a wonderfully dusky smell.

At weekends and in the long summer evenings we visited the beauty spots, the villages and coastal towns that surrounded Hull: Bridlington, Sunk Island, Spurn Point, Flamborough Head, the Wolds. On one of these trips – to the seaside town of Withernsea – David took his first steps unaided. He was about one year old. I remember it vividly. He wore a white fur one-piece suit, which Jean had sent from Canada, and a little hat. He looked so bonny.

Mr Priestman leased a wooden bungalow in the middle of a six acre field near the sea at Ulrome, a small village on the coast about forty minutes' drive from Hull.

During the summer he used to run a boys' Christian holiday camp there and Douglas had usually helped out in the years before and after the war. In the spring of 1953, when David was about eighteen months, Mr Priestman asked if we would like to use it as a holiday home in return for cleaning and airing it and generally preparing things for the camp.

We thought it an excellent idea, especially as we had little money to spend on a holiday. But it called for hard work.

The bungalow had to be cleaned

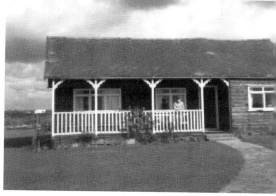

Penn Cottage at Ulrome

throughout and all the bedding aired. Douglas opened up the outbuildings, cleared out layers of bird droppings, and got the cooking ranges working, and I washed sheets and tablecloths. Meanwhile David played on the lawn in the sunshine.

Douglas erected fences and dug latrines. Instead of flush toilets we had Elsans. Every few days Douglas had the unpleasant job of emptying them in a deep hole he had dug in the ground – a long way from the house. The bungalow had no mod cons: no electricity or mains gas; no phone, of course; there were paraffin lamps to provide light in the evenings, Calor gas for cooking, and an open wood fire for heating. Water had to be heated either in a kettle or, for washing clothes, in a large copper. There was running water, but we preferred to use rainwater from the butt outside for baths and washing. It was soft and pure, and left hair feeling clean and smooth.

Staying at Ulrome made such a change from city life, and it was such fun. Whenever we could, we ate outside in the open country air, and our meals included fresh eggs and milk from the nearby farm.

I soon wanted another child. Douglas was afraid to let me. There was a lot of discussion at the time about Down's syndrome. It had recently been linked to older parents. I had been forty-three when David was born. I was now forty-five. Douglas was fifty-one. But I had never thought about my age for one moment. I had passed an easy pregnancy and the birth was without complications. David was a healthy, bouncing boy and I was very happy with him.

David says he can actually remember the time, when he was barely two, that I asked him if he wanted a little sister. He gave it a moment's thought. He was probably thinking about what he would have to give up, what he would have to share. Then he shook his head and quite categorically said, 'No.'

Despite Douglas and David's reservations, I made an appointment to see Dr Winchester. 'I want another child,' I explained, 'but my husband is afraid to let me have one. I want a girl,' I went on. 'I've got a lovely boy. I want a girl now.'

'Well, I can't tell you if you'll have a girl,' he said. 'But I'll be able to tell you if you can have another child.'

After he had examined me he said, 'There's no reason medically why you should not have another child. Ask your husband to come in and see me.'

'He won't come, I can tell you that now,' I said. 'He's very much against my having another child. But I'm sure everything would be fine. I had a good pregnancy, didn't I? And I've been very fit.'

'Well, if you can get him to come and see me, it would be a help to you both, I'm sure.'

But it was as I feared. Douglas refused to go. So I had to give up the idea of another child.

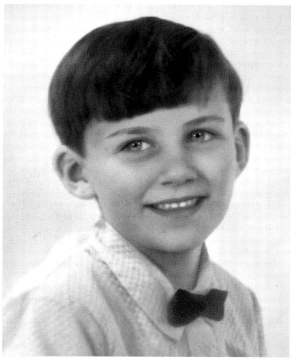

David at five years old

13

Sister Tutor

My teaching is not mine, but His who sent me
John 7.16

When David was barely two, the Western General Hospital approached me about when I might be able to start as sister tutor at the school. Fortunately, I was able to find a pre-nursery place for David in a large house off Pearson Park, which was just five minutes' walk from Eldon Grove.

Working at the Western General School of Nursing was a source of great joy and satisfaction. I was responsible for the training of pre-nursing students as well as those taking the full nursing course. The schoolrooms were part of the old hospital, and were well-equipped with a lecture theatre where I could show slides and films, a demonstration room which was set out like a small hospital ward, and a kitchen area for the teaching of domestic hygiene. Though it was near the centre of the city, the Western General had the feel of a cottage hospital. At the front, where we looked out on to Anlaby Road, there were shrubs and trees and raised flower beds. Behind us in the quadrant was a pretty little walled garden.

As part of the course I arranged trips to the local companies and utilities connected with the work of a nurse. With each new intake of students there would be the visit to Reckitt's to see the manufacture of various drugs and antiseptic creams and bandages. We would each be given little sample boxes to take away with us. The local chocolate manufacturer was Needler, and we would witness the measures taken to ensure hygiene in the preparation and packing of the various products, before coming away with complimentary selection boxes and bars of chocolate. However, whenever we paid a call on the local Water Board to see how they dealt with our sewage, we were always happy to leave empty-handed!

I loved the teaching, and all the many girls – and the few male trainees – who passed through my school.

* * *

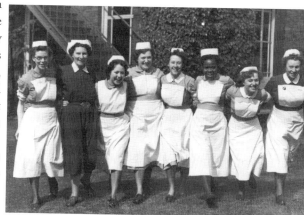

In the gardens of Western General Hospital with my students

Douglas had a cousin in Birmingham called Albert Banks. Brother to cousin Charlie who lived in Cleethorpes, Albert had been headmaster of the Harborne Collegiate School. When he retired in the mid-Fifties, he decided not to give up teaching – which was his passion – but to open a private school where children who had experienced educational difficulties of one sort or another could receive high-quality personal tuition.

He found a large detached house in one of the outlying districts of Birmingham called Kings Norton. Gradually he built up a fine reputation. His small school would take in a range of pupils from the age of nine to seventeen. There would never be more than about twenty pupils at any one time, and the entire group was coached in the same classroom. Albert believed that the mix of ages and experience was a valuable part of his pupils' education.

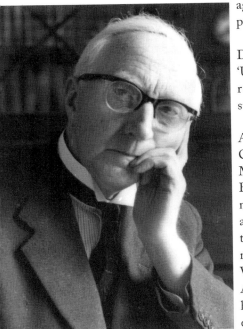

Albert Banks

He was a dear man, and exceptionally clever. David took to him at once and called him 'Uncle' Albert. It was probably Albert's wide-ranging love of literature and science that stimulated David's interests in these subjects.

On one of the early occasions that we visited Albert at the Manor School, I remembered that Captain Giles, who had brought me home from Malta during the war, lived in a district of Birmingham called Edgbaston. I looked up his name in the Birmingham telephone directory, and there it was. I phoned the number and spoke to Mrs Giles. She was delighted to hear from me, and I made arrangements to call.

We drove across to Edgbaston – Douglas, Albert, David and I – and found the house. It had been fifteen years since Gilo and I had seen each other. He was in his seventies, a fine-looking man still, but long since retired from the Navy. Soon after landing at the Clyde in 1942 he was ordered back to sea on another war mission. His ship was attacked and he was severely injured. He was subsequently decorated by the Queen.

After lunch, we went on an excursion to the nearby town of Warwick to see the historic castle. Standing on the bridge overlooking the castle moat, Gilo described to Douglas and Albert something of what it was like on that journey back from Malta. When he got to the part where he had taken me up on deck to see the sailors and the Admiral of the Fleet on the Ark Royal, I expressed my disbelief as I had all those years ago. But he said to them, 'It really was in her honour, you know. She won't believe me, but it really was.'

I suddenly realised that Gilo had not been teasing me about the Admiral's message after all.

Albert invited the Giles family for a meal with us later that week, and from that time on he and the captain became good friends. Gilo, his mischievous sense of humour undimmed, took to referring to Albert as 'Mr Chips'.

By 1956 I was Secretary of the Hull branch of the College of Nursing. The branch was informed that two thousand nurses were to be chosen from hospitals all over the world to attend the Eleventh Quadrennial Congress of the International Council of Nurses which was to take place in Rome in May and June 1957. Our branch had been selected to send one of our nurses, and the person who was chosen would be the branch representive at the congress. Who that representative would be was to be decided fairly and impartially by arranging a draw.

It was a simple affair. A number of raffle tickets, one for each of us, was put into a hat and we all took it in turns to pick one out. I drew the marked ticket and was thereby chosen to visit Rome as the representative of the nurses of Hull.

I had to travel to London for the first leg of the trip. There I met up with the other representatives from Great Britain. We were given a lavish buffet reception over which the Queen Mother presided. Afterwards we were to have the honour of being presented to her.

I was fascinated to be so close to a royal figure. During the buffet, as we were all eating, I could not take my eyes off her. She ate her food with her gloves on, I noticed, and so did her lady-in-waiting, except that her gloves exposed the tips of her fingers. There were several gentlemen walking about, keeping their eye on us. Some sort of security men, I imagine. One of them must have noticed that I was staring at the Queen Mother. He came over and put his mouth to my ear.

'Stop watching her,' he said in a low, rather menacing voice. 'She has to eat her refreshments as well as you.'

The journey was to be overland by coach and train. We left from Victoria coach station and, once in France, we travelled by train. Arriving in Rome, it came home to me how exciting it was to be part of such a large enterprise. The mix of nurses was truly international. Each day we were picked up by car from our various hotels to attend the lectures and conferences. The congress took place in a massive building which was one of the last that Mussolini had built before his demise. As part of the opening ceremony we each had to carry a flag, denoting the country and area we were representing, and march around the huge indoor stadium.

Then we were invited to the Vatican. I learned that it is the smallest independent state in the world, no more than one hundred acres in size, and yet contains some of the finest art treasures in the world.

It was a hot day. First we wandered around the Vatican Gardens and the Belvedere Park, before ending up at the square outside St Peter's Church and the papal palace. There were crowds of people packed together, all standing waiting for Pope Pius XII to emerge on the balcony. But we were ushered inside the palace. No one was allowed to take cameras inside, and people were asked to take their shoes off.

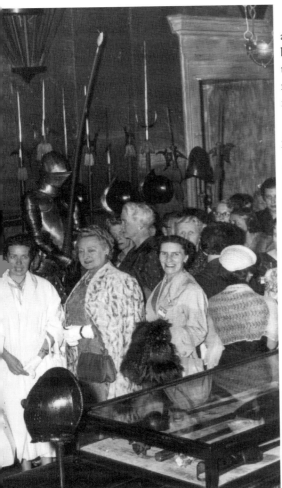
The International Congress of Nurses, Rome

We waited for an age. Eventually he appeared. He was carried in on a chair by six men dressed in ordinary suits and ties, which looked odd given the fine robes the Pope was wearing and the medieval opulence of the Vatican.

He held out his hands to us all and gave his blessing in six different languages. Women with babies were holding them out to be blessed. It was so hot in there and there were so many of us that people were starting to faint. It was mostly the nurses who seemed to be affected.

Every night there was a different activity as part of the international congress. One night, for example, there was a concert of madrigals. Another night, some of the nurses sang their national songs, dressed in national costume. We did not wear our nursing uniform while we were there, since we were not on duty. I wore what I often wore when teaching, a maroon dress held in at the waist by a belt with a solid silver clasp in the shape of two interconnecting fish to denote my star sign, Pisces.

At the famous fountain of Trevi, we all threw our coins into the water and made our secret wishes. Mine was – I can tell it now – that one day my husband and son would come back with me to Rome. Sadly, my wish was never granted.

I was away for six weeks altogether. After the congress was finished we visited Venice. Up until that time the weather had been perfect. Blue skies, no rain. When we got to Venice, it poured down. But it was still beautiful, especially the Lido and the palaces. At night we were taken by gondola along the canals. It all looked very beautiful, but the smell was awful. The canals were like open drains, and people would just throw their garbage into the water.

On our return journey we also called at Naples and Assisi. At Assisi we saw the crypt where St Francis was buried. It was full of monuments to him. We imagined there would be much wild life in the area. Strangely, there was not a bird or animal to be seen.

The Leeds branch of the College of Nursing had sent me £10 to spend on the trip, on condition that I gave them a talk about it when I returned. £10 was a substantial amount of money – equal to £200 or £300 in today's money – and it made things a lot easier. I was able to buy little gifts for Douglas and David. And giving the talk, I knew, would pose no difficulties. There was so much to tell.

1961 was a year for renewing old acquaintances. The first reunion was with Eric Doyle. He was now Professor of Paediatrics at Dublin University. We had exchanged the occasional letter and card over the years, but it had been fifteen years since we had last seen each other, when I was matron at Barnardo's.

An opportunity arose to visit Ireland. Ruth Joelson, Granny Joelson's daughter, had married an Irish bible student called Jim Craig and they had gone out on mission work together to Beirut in the Lebanon. Back on furlough, they had stayed for a time in my old flat downstairs and we came to know them as valued friends. Jim had relations in Bangor and they invited us for a holiday – to see something of Ireland, north and south. I let Eric know that we were to be over there during the summer, and he replied saying we must call on him in Dublin.

He met us at the station, driving up in a plush green sports car, a Sunbeam Rapier, which very much impressed Douglas and David. He had become extremely distinguished-looking, hair greying at the temples, and was as charming as ever: softly spoken, courteous and considerate. Bringing out a box of chocolates for me and a box of sweets for David, he took us into the city, showed us his surgery and then drove us through the Wicklow hills to lunch in a beautiful country restaurant. David took to him at once, and he chatted away to Douglas, but I was aware of a slight distance, a kind of formality, between the two of us. Strange to say, I think it was shyness on both sides.

It was not until we had sat down to the meal that the situation changed dramatically. He asked me to pass over a dish of steaming vegetables. I did so, but the dish slipped from my grasp, carrots and broccoli cascading down into his lap. David roared with laughter – and so, I'm thankful to say, did Eric. After that, the ice was well and truly broken!

The second reunion of the year turned out to be a unique celebration. My sister Jean had decided to come over and see the family again. She left her husband and her son Brythan behind in Canada. Douglas, David and I drove down to Heathrow airport to meet her in. She was coming back to stay with us in Hull, from where we were to take her to visit relations in Wales. But first, the big event: a coming together of all the surviving Staerck family members – Albert, Alice, Jean, Mary, Eddie and myself – for what must have been the first time since the family was broken up in the early years of the century.

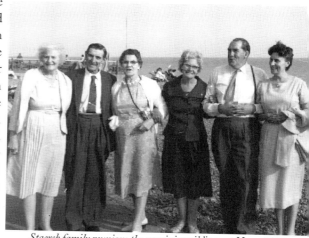

Staerck family reunion: the surviving siblings at Hove, 1961

William had died in 1944. We all met up at Mary and Frank's house in Hove. Other members of the family were present: Margaret and Fred Samuels and their son Colin, who was the same age as David, and their little daughter Helen; Alice's husband, Norman Pluck; Eddie's wife and daughters. It was an extraordinary get-together, and, sadly, was to prove a once-in-a-lifetime event.

The third renewing of old acquaintance could not be called a reunion. It was more a reminder. I was in hospital having a routine operation and happened to see in *Nursing Mirror* a piece about the Reverend Eric Wells, of whom I had heard nothing since before the war. Dorothy had died and he had married Hilda de Pinto, who had just retired after fourteen years as matron of the Princess Alice Memorial and St Mary's Hospitals, Eastbourne. The item described how they first met in the early years of the war when Hilda had been a sister, and Eric the hospital chaplain, at Pembury Hospital, Kent. My godson, John Wells, had acted as best man.

I wrote to Eric congratulating him and wishing him every happiness, and promptly received a warm reply in which he gave me news of John:

South Bersted Vicar Weds In Secret

THE date and place of the wedding of the Rev. Eric Wells, Vicar of South Bersted, was a well-kept secret.

On Monday, at St Richard's Church, Aldwick, he was married to Miss Hilda de Pinto, until recently Matron of Eastbourne General Hospitals, and few knew about it.

The service was conducted by the Bishop of Chichester (Dr. Roger Wilson), assisted by the Vicar of Aldwick (Canon H. Tarrant).

Mr. John Wells, the son of the bridegroom, who has just joined the staff of Eton College, was best man.

The bride was given away by Dr. E. D. Grasby, Medical Superintendent of the County Hospital, Pembury, an old friend of the bride and bridegroom.

It was while a sister at that hospital and when the bridegroom was hospital chaplain there that they first met.

… After leaving Eastbourne College, he did his National Service as a 2nd Lieutenant in the Royal Sussex Regiment and served for a year in Korea. On demobilisation in Sept, 1957, he went up to Oxford on an Open Scholarship. After a year there, he was picked to spend a year in Germany and went to Munich in Sept. '58. In 1959, he returned to Oxford and finished his time there in June of this year. Then of all things, he was offered a job on the teaching staff at Eton where he is now teaching French and German. All the way through, he has been the best of sons, and in regard to my second marriage, he took to Hilda immediately and she to him.

As to ourselves, we are settled in the friendliest and busiest of Parishes. Everybody is kindness itself; the work is enormously encouraging; and our Bishop (who, of course, is only some 6 miles from here) is the best friend any man ever had.

Hilda joins me in wishing you a good recovery and all the very best to your son and husband…

In the early 1960s there was a huge reorganisation of the Health Service. The Western General Hospital was going to be pulled down to make room for a larger hospital, a fourteen-storey building which was to be known as the Hull Royal Infirmary. We were sad to lose our little school, but a larger one was to be built in its place – a major teaching centre for the area. There was no doubt about the prestige it was intended the new school should command. But one question remained. Who would be running it? Who was to be appointed principal?

An advert appeared for the post of Principal of the Hull Royal Infirmary School of Nursing. Applications were invited from those with the appropriate qualifications and experience. I had been the principal sister tutor at the Western General School since 1953. But the new school that was under construction was going to be much larger and more important – the major nurses' training establishment for our part of the country. My own position would not survive the relocation, though I naturally hoped to be reappointed as one of the tutors in the new school.

I knew of at least two people who were in line for becoming principal of the new school, both of them with greater claim to it, I felt, than I. There was the principal tutor from Kingston General Hospital, Mr Bob Reeve; and then there was the favourite for the job, since she was already principal of the existing Hull Royal Hospital School of Nursing. Her name was Miss Close. The post had been advertised to comply with the procedural rules, but it seemed clear that this was a formality and that the job was hers but in name. Nevertheless, I felt it would be wrong not to apply, and in due course an appointment was arranged for me to attend an interview before the hospital committee at the Hull Royal.

On the appointed day I left my teaching duties, put on my hat and coat, and caught the bus for the Hull Royal. On arrival I was taken up to the committee room. Miss Close and Mr Reeve were already there, sitting outside in the corridor. We waited for what seemed like an age. Then Miss Close was asked in, while Mr Reeve and I continued to wait for what seemed like another age. Then it was my turn. I held out no expectations. From what Miss Close had been saying as we had waited together, she was certain she was the one for the job.

I was asked all sorts of questions. Why did I think I was right for the job? I wasn't entirely sure that I was. Shouldn't the Western General have been training pupil nurses? No, I didn't think so. Why not? Because Kingston General had been set up to train pupil nurses and had instructors for this purpose. So, at the Western General, we had been free to train probationers to become State Registered Nurses.

The line of questioning was pursued until the committee seemed to have formed an impression of me. Then it was time to wait outside again, and Mr Reeve went in to be interviewed. When they were done with him, we were asked to wait for a further period while the committee deliberated over their decision.

They were such a long time I got tired of sitting there. I had work to get on with back at the school and saw no point in hanging on. I was sure Miss Close had got the post. It was all cut and dried. I got my hat and coat and left.

When I got back to the Western General the assistant matron came across to see me – to find out, I imagined, how I had got on. 'What's happened?' she asked.

'I don't know,' I said. 'I didn't stay around to find out. I think Miss Close must have got it.'

'No,' she said, 'I mean what's happened to you. They're all wondering. Apparently, they came out to call you back in for another chat but you'd already gone.'

'Yes, well, they'll have already decided who they want, I'm sure. They don't need to see me again.'

'I don't think so,' she said. 'They want to arrange another appointment with you. And this time I'm coming with you to make sure you stay.'

So, a week later, the assistant matron accompanied me to yet another interview. I was beginning to feel a little nervous about it all now. When we got there, Mr Reeve was waiting again, along with a lady who was a sister tutor from somewhere else – not in the Hull District at all – who had also applied for the post. There was no sign of Miss Close.

The same process was followed. The same questions were asked, and there were the same lengthy periods of waiting outside. The committee seemed keen to impress upon me that the posts of principal and deputy principal were still open. They referred to rumours to the contrary and wanted to assure me that these were entirely without foundation.

The next morning Miss Close came into my office. She wanted me to hand over all my books, my register of student nurses and so on.

'No, I can't let you have those. Why should you want them?'

'Well, as I'm the principal now, I must have access to these things.'

I thought she was probably right, especially as I hadn't seen her at the second interview, but felt I should wait for the official announcement. She started trying to pull rank and to throw her weight about, but I stuck by what I had said and refused to be intimidated.

Somehow, the girls – my students – got to hear about what was happening. Before long there was a queue stretching from my office to the matron's office.

'We're going to see matron,' they told me. 'We're not going to have Miss Close as our principal. We'll resign if she takes over.'

After they had taken their grievances to matron, she called me in to talk about it. 'What can I do?' she asked.

'They do seem absolutely determined to resign if Miss Close gets the job,' I replied, 'and I must say I feel like that, too.'

'Why?'

'Well, the first thing that woman did was to come round and ask for all my books. She was throwing her weight about, saying she was the principal and that I was subordinate to her.'

Matron sighed. 'Oh, well, I'll have to see them again and try to mollify them somehow. The absurd thing is that nothing's decided yet. You do know that, don't you?'

'Well, that's what the committee tells me.'

'I have it on the best authority that they've not yet made up their mind. Even if she is to get the job, Miss Close is behaving quite wrongly.'

Matron called a meeting with the nurses and explained that the matter wasn't altogether settled yet, but that for the moment, since Miss Close was principal at the Hull Royal, they should do as she said and save their protests until they knew who was to be principal of the new school.

Miss Close herself did not feel it necessary to wait. She started to interview the nurses, and there were several she said she would not have in her school. She claimed, quite wrongly in my opinion, that they were not fit to be nurses.

There were twin sisters in the school, Margaret and Marjorie Hindmarsh. They were good little cadets. During their interview, Miss Close asked them about their mother, and discovered that she suffered rather badly from ill-health. She responded by telling them that they had no place training to be nurses; they should be at home nursing their mother. These two

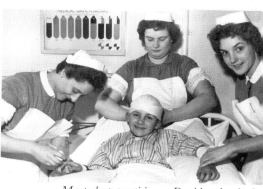

My students practising on David at the school

delightful girls were duly entered on Miss Close's list of nurses whom she would not take into her school.

Naturally, they were deeply upset. They came to me – Margaret and Marjorie – and told me all about it. They were promising students, I told them, and in my view would make excellent nurses. But all we could do was to sit it out and wait for the committee to reach its decision. I gave them a test to gauge their progress in a way that I could formally present to Miss Close. As I expected, they did extremely well. As it turned out they both continued their training and won qualifications as SRN and SEN respectively.

A third interview was called by the committee. Again, Mr Reeve and I were present, as was the other woman who it turned out was from some other northern hospital district. There was the same performance of waiting, and questions, and then more waiting, and more questions. This time, when they asked if I had anything I wanted to bring up before they made their final choice, I said I had. 'I just want you to know that the school means a lot to me. It's a good and important school and I want the best for it, and the highest standard for the nurses. Whoever is chosen, I shall do my utmost to help and support them.' And with that I left.

This time when the assistant matron came to see how I got on, I said, 'I didn't get it.' I knew I hadn't.

'Oh, well. Never mind,' she said consolingly.

The next morning a letter arrived from the chairman of the committee, Mr Bates. I was right. I had not got the job of principal. But neither had Miss Close. It had gone to Mr Reeve.

Since I had no expectation of the post, I could only feel relief and grateful surprise that the shadow of Miss Close had been removed from my nurses and the school. But the letter went on to say that they wished to appoint me deputy principal. A couple of days later Mr Bates rang me up and asked me to call at his office.

'You know, it wasn't all cut and dried,' he said when I got there. 'We were most impressed with you, especially at the last meeting. In the end we felt that the post of deputy is the one closest to your experience as sister tutor. Mr Reeve will actually have a great deal of administrative responsibility to occupy him. In effect, the day-to-day teaching and running of the school will be down to you.

You'll have your own office and you'll have equal say with Mr Reeve in selecting the applicants for intake each year. Are you in a position to accept our offer?'

I said I was.

'There is one other thing which, now you are his deputy, you might help us with,' he went on. I couldn't think what he might be going say. 'Will you ask Mr Reeve to wear a white shirt and sensible tie – black or navy blue. He's not presentable enough. He needs to smarten up. Will you do that for me?'

'I'll try,' I said.

The next day I received another letter from Mr Bates:

> The committee asked me to explain to you that the appointment of one person to take charge is really a question of *primus inter pares* and I have no doubt that you appreciate the fact that as deputy you will have a very major role to play and one which I am sure you will enjoy.

I was not sure what *primus inter pares* meant. I asked Douglas, and he looked it up for me at the back of a dictionary.

'First among equals,' he said.

The day came when work on demolition began. Seeing the old school coming down was terrible. It was like having my teeth pulled, it meant so much to me. The schooling of the nurses had to go on, of course, and we did the best we could by relocating temporarily to Landsdown House, which was the nurses' home for the old Western General.

All the nurses who had trained and worked at the Western General were terribly upset to see it go. In a funny way, the act of destroying the building actually pulled them all closer together. They remembered those special days and wanted some means of keeping the memory alive, and of keeping in touch as their various careers took them away from Hull and each other.

As a member of the General Nursing Council I used to go to all the major hospitals in the UK to act as examiner. At this time of reorganisation I happened

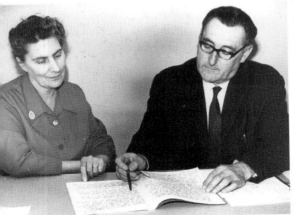

to speak to a senior member of the Council and mentioned the nurses' desire to keep in touch, and she suggested that we might try starting some kind of society, a league of former students. So I put a notice in the *Hull Daily Mail* for anyone who had trained or taught or worked at the old Western General Hospital, inviting them to attend a meeting at a certain date and time and at such-and-such a place to discuss forming a League of Friends.

Checking exam papers with Mr Reeve

On the night we were not expecting many – our faith was so low – but a hundred and seventy people turned up! I put to them the advice I had received from the General Nursing Council and there was immediate approval of the idea. That night we formed a committee. I was elected chairman. Marianne Tansey, a colleague and friend, was made secretary, and we also appointed a treasurer. Then we decided on the frequency of our future meetings and what our society would try to accomplish. We did not want the League to be a purely nostalgic and social association, so a yearly project which would in some way help others was agreed upon.

That first year we contacted the Hull Social Services for a list of people who might be in need at Christmas and set out to provide hampers of food and provisions for them. During the year our members set aside one or two items each week from their shopping excursions for the hamper project. Others who were good at knitting made hundreds of knitted squares which were sewn together into blankets or rugs.

As Christmas approached we assembled a huge pile of groceries. We spent a whole evening dividing up the supplies and packing them into the hampers, which we lined with red or blue tissue paper. Each hamper had a Christmas pudding, a Christmas cake, mince pies, a quarter of tea, coffee, a box of dates and many other items that we took for granted at Christmas but which those who were to receive the hampers could ill afford.

Our League of Friends is still an active force today, and in 1991 we celebrated its Silver Jubilee.

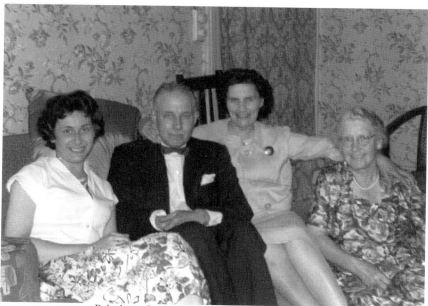

Relaxing at home with Joan Peers and Marjorie Beevers

14

A New School

Therefore we will not fear though the earth should change,
though the mountains shake in the heart of the sea
Psalms 46.2

Eventually the old Western General was entirely demolished and work was begun on the new hospital. In 1966 we were invited to be present at the laying of the foundation stone. Anthony Eden, the former prime minister, presided over the ceremony.

Storey by storey, the new Hull Royal Infirmary rose, until one day Douglas and I were able to travel in a fast lift right to the newly completed roof and take photographs from the top. The view across the city was breathtaking.

The hospital was going to be officially opened by the Queen. We were all very excited as the day approached. A big marquee was put up in the grounds and I was invited, along with other senior members of the hospital, to attend as a guest at the opening ceremony. I took Douglas's cine camera to take pictures of the cavalcade as it arrived.

We were ushered into the marquee and took our places on chairs newly upholstered in pink and yellow and white. Then the Queen came in. As she walked down between the two blocks of seats she looked so small, and very neat, in a navy dress with hat to match, and her complexion – she passed very near to me so I got a good view of her face – was flawless. She looked so young and beautiful.

She signed the official book and said a few words, then declared the Hull Royal Infirmary open, and asked God's blessing on it.

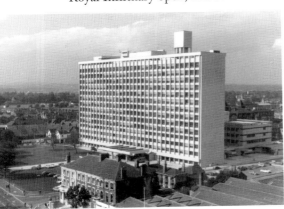

After she had left, we were invited back to the new nurses' home where a special tea was waiting for us. We chatted away, full of the novelty of seeing the Queen at such close quarters. Before the ceremony, she had been taken around the hospital and had talked to the patients and staff, who were now buzzing with excitement and pleasure.

At last we were able to move from the cramped conditions at Landsdown House to the new school of nursing

The Hull Royal Infirmary, newly built

which, though not as pretty as the old school, was purpose-built for the training of nurses and equipped with the latest teaching aids. It had been built in the shadow of the towering new hospital, well back from the busy main road – not far from the new helicopter landing pad designed to fly in emergency cases – and just across the way from Casualty and Emergency Admissions.

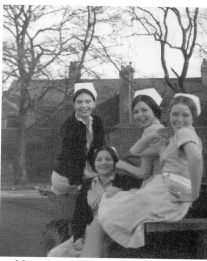

The two-storey building was small enough to feel homely. Yet its rooms were spacious, filled with light and air. I had to unpack crates and crates of teaching materials, and boxes and boxes of books, epidiascope, slide projector and so forth. Everything was new and of the very best quality. No expense had been spared to establish the Hull School of Nursing as a model of its kind.

My students in the grounds of the new school

There were study rooms and classrooms, a lecture room and library, a rest room and offices for the tutors. I had my own, very pleasant office, with large windows which looked on to grass and newly-planted trees and shrubs, as well as several mature trees which had survived the years of demolition and building work. Mr Reeve and I got down to the business of choosing the next year's intake of students and started interviewing them together.

Since he delegated much of the teaching work to me, I found that my new job as deputy principal was very similar to that of sister tutor at the Western General and soon discovered I was enjoying my new position every bit as much. For the next seven years I was happy in my work – very happy indeed.

For a long time I had promised myself that I would learn to drive. Along with my work at the school, I was still touring the country, examining for the General Nursing Council. The idea of being able to drive to some of these places, as well as to the school every day, was a powerful incentive to take the lessons. But I kept putting it off, partly because of pressure of work, but mainly because I was afraid of being behind the wheel. Now and then, when we were on some isolated stretch of road, I would swap places with Douglas, and he would try to teach me. It was not an ideal way to learn. He would get agitated if I crunched the gears, and I would be petrified if I saw so much as a bicycle approaching a hundred yards away. So, once I was settled into the new job, I decided to book some lessons.

To my surprise, learning to drive came relatively easily, and far from being afraid I thoroughly enjoyed the sensation of being in the driving seat. The trouble was that I became extremely nervous when taking the test, with the result that I failed – several times. I prayed and prayed that the Lord would help me through, but my nervousness always caused me to make silly mistakes.

As a small girl at school, my ears had once been inexpertly syringed by a nurse, with the result that my right eardrum was perforated – to this day I vividly remember the sudden bang it produced – and I lost the ability to hear with that ear. I had to be careful to keep water from getting in my ear whenever I swam, otherwise it would cause me excruciating pain. But however careful I was, from time to time an infection would develop and I would have to seek immediate medical help.

On one occasion, the infection was so bad that I had to be admitted to the new Hull Royal to have special antibiotic treatment administered over a ten-day period. The treatment included antibiotic eardrops, regular injections, and a penicillin drip. I was thoroughly infused with drugs. It was this event that had a significant bearing on my final driving test.

The day of my discharge from hospital happened to coincide with the day of my latest driving test. I could have changed the date, but that would have meant waiting another six months. I wanted to get the thing over with. As she signed my discharge papers, the sister warned me that the effect of the treatment might continue to make me feel drowsy for the next day or two. I said nothing about my impending driving test and on leaving the hospital went straight to the British School of Motoring offices, where the examiner was waiting for me beside the car he was to test me in. We got into the car and off I drove.

Instead of being racked with nerves I was perfectly calm. It felt like a real answer to my prayer. To my surprise I was rather enjoying the experience of driving through the city traffic. As he guided me through the back streets of Old Hull the examiner didn't say much but I felt I was doing all the right things. Eventually we came back up George Street. The road was lined with cars parked on both sides. Opposite the shop called Carmichael's, the examiner said to me, 'See, there's a car just about to move out from its parking position. I want you to move in front of that space, reverse into it and park.'

Reverse parking was my least favourite aspect of driving. I inched forward as the other car drove off. The space it had left looked very tiny to me, and I wasn't at all certain I'd be able to manoeuvre my way into it. Fortunately – and I'm sure this was an answer to prayer – at that very moment I noticed that the car parked in front was also leaving. I waited calmly until it had gone and then to my great relief positioned the car more or less faultlessly in the ample parking space.

'Now, Mrs Banks,' said the examiner, 'drive out again, turn around so that we are facing the opposite direction, and we'll go back to the office.'

I dreaded the Three Point Turn but that's what he was asking me to do. Again to my surprise, I managed to carry out the tricky manoeuvre without the usual jolting and juddering and bumping of tyres on the pavement and we were back at the BSM office in no time. The examiner solemnly filled in his examination report and then looked across at me.

'Well, congratulations, Mrs Banks. You've done it.'

'Really?' I said. 'I don't believe it.'

'Does it come as a surprise?'

'Yes, it does rather.'

'Well, it shouldn't. You were in control at all times. A very good performance.'

'Oh, how marvellous!' I said. It was finally sinking in that I would have to take no more driving lessons – or tests for that matter. 'Then it's an answer to prayer.'

'Well, whatever it was, congratulations. You did well.'

'I've been in hospital for ten days,' I said, 'and I was only discharged today. I've been rather pumped up with drugs, I'm afraid.'

'Well, I can't say that I approve of drugs, but that must have had a bearing on it. I've never had such a calm examinee.'

I knew, however, that really it was an answer to prayer. How delighted I was as I made my way home. It was just after lunchtime but Douglas had come home from work and waited for me to see how I had got on. It was wonderful to be able to share this news with him. We rejoiced together.

Not long after, my brother Eddie became seriously ill. His daughter Peggy, who was a nurse, rang me with the news.

'Auntie Mina, if you want to see Dad, you'd better come straightaway. He's sinking into unconsciousness.'

Though we had been able to see very little of each other over the years, we were always close. He had not been stationed long in York and about ten years before he had moved with his family to London. I went down at once.

His condition was extremely grave. He was suffering the final painful stages of lung cancer. Within a few hours of my arriving, he died. My favourite brother. The one who had given me my name.

Eddie left three grown-up daughters. His house and possessions were to be sold and the money divided between them. One of his possessions was his dear little car, a black Morris Minor, registration number 50 MPJ.

For a time after passing my test it had been no problem to use our white Morris traveller whenever I needed it. But as I had begun to drive the car more, we realised that I really needed one for myself. Now I saw it would mean so much to me if I could buy Eddie's Morris Minor.

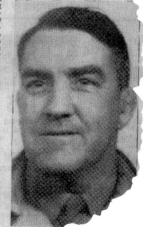

Surrey Comet, Saturday, July 29, 1967.

C.D. leader dies day after retiring

MR. A. E. STAERCK, ex-Army officer and Esher's Civil Defence leader for 10 years, died suddenly + his home on Tuesday, his 65th birthday and one day ˆer he officially retired from his post.

ˌis colleagues in the close-knit her unit had been preparing surprise for him—a special presentation of his long service ˌedal for 15 years in the corps.

An official tribute from the Civil Defence Committee on the occasion of his retirement appears ˌn the minutes to go before Esher Council next week.

On Wednesday, the Clek to the council (Mr. A. G. Chamberlin) expressed the feelings of the council officers. "This is very sad news to us all. We have lost an excellent man.

"He was an absolutely firstlass officer and it was due entirely to his leadership, keenness and sincere belief in the work of ˌivil Defence and the necessity ˌr it, that the Esher unit reached ˌh a high level of efficiency."

HIGH REGARD

ˌen and women of the unit ˌ whom was his youngest Pamela, now 27, and ˌars' service in the ˌ regard for the

Returning to Hull I mentioned my idea to Douglas. He looked up the value of Eddie's car. £250 seemed a fair price. The family accepted my offer and a few days later I caught the train down to London for Eddie's funeral, having arranged to drive back in his little black car of which I was now the proud and excited owner.

Eddie had been an extremely competent driver. He had passed the advanced driving test and there was an attractive Advanced Driver's metal badge fixed to the radiator grille. As Peggy was removing Eddie's belongings from the car I pointed to the grille.

'Let me keep that badge on there,' I said.

'But you're not an advanced driver.'

'No, I know. But just for memory's sake. I'd like it.'

So it remained, fixed in place on the radiator.

I left at six in the morning. I had not so far driven the car any real distance. Now it had to take me all the way back to Hull. Peggy's husband Tom set off in front of me and led me to the nearest motorway. Once there, he signalled that he was turning off. Then I was on my own. It was the first time I had been on a motorway with nobody else in the car, but on that journey down the M1 I was so happy. I felt such release. I was singing at the top of my voice. If anyone had heard me they would have thought me mad. But elation was flooding through me. I was sure that Eddie was sitting beside me. It was a wonderful feeling.

I was not far from Hull when suddenly there was a banging noise which seemed to be coming from the engine. Luckily, I saw a garage and pulled into it. A man had a look under the bonnet and found a screw had worked its way loose, causing the carburettor to rattle. He adjusted something and told me that it would get me home all right, but that it should be checked over properly in a day or two.

I continued on my way and was soon home. There was a note waiting for me from Douglas, welcoming me back and reminding me that he had a dental appointment. I rang the dentist to let Douglas know I had arrived back safely. They were just about to drill his tooth when the dental nurse passed on the message.

'Oh, that's marvellous,' he said. 'I didn't expect her so soon. She's driven up from London,' he told them proudly. 'On her own!'

That little Morris Minor was such a lovely little car. I called it Ebenezer because it was black as ebony. More than anything, I enjoyed the independence it gave me. I drove to the school every day and took it examining. It was such a help. I used to take David to school and then go on to the Hull Royal. One day, driving down Beverley Road, the noise recurred. As I turned into Anlaby Road, nearing the hospital, I saw a garage.

Two young men came out to look at the car. 'This is a giggle,' said one.

'You need a new coil,' said the other.

'How much is that?' I asked.

'Oh, that'd be about two quid, at least,' he said. 'But we haven't got one here. You'll have to go up Pickering Road to get it.'

'How am I going to get up there? I'm meant to be lecturing all day today. And I don't have any money with me – not so much as that anyhow.'

'I don't know, lady. But that's what you'll need to get it going again.'

At that moment, a young man walked into the garage. I recognised him as John from the admin department of the hospital. I called over to him.

He saw me and came over. I explained my predicament and asked if he could help. He said at once, 'Yes, Mrs Banks, I'll go and pick it up for you. I've got my car here. That's no problem.'

After they fixed the coil, I had no more trouble with Ebenezer for years.

Auntie Dagmar was now living in Cheam in London. She had recently celebrated her eightieth birthday. In the years since Douglas and I were married, she had increasingly come under the influence of Bob Hutchinson, who was now managing all her affairs, and though I tried to keep in contact with her, I felt more and more excluded. It seemed that Bob Hutchinson's relations and friends were taking over her life.

Whenever I had the opportunity – for example, when I was examining in the London area – I would go round and see her, taking some little gift or flowers. Once, not long after her birthday, I was down in London examining at St Thomas's Hospital. Having a few hours to spare I decided to go round and see her.

A middle-aged woman I did not recognise opened the door and eyed me suspiciously. When I asked to see Mrs André, she told me that would not be possible. I tried to explain who I was, but to no avail. 'You can't come in,' she said, and was about to close the door. But I was worried by this time, so I pushed through and went straight to Auntie's room.

Auntie's eyes lit up when she saw me. She wasn't able to get up from her chair but she greeted me warmly, giving me a big hug and telling the woman who I was and that she could leave us together.

I was shocked at Auntie's appearance. She looked flushed and there was a look of anxiety in her eyes. At the same time there were symptoms of over-sedation.

'Who is that woman?' I asked, trying to keep my voice low.

'That's matron,' she replied. 'She looks after me now, dear. Bob arranged it.'

'Matron? Matron of where?'

'I'm not sure. That's what she said I should call her. She came over from Cardiff. She was matron there, I think. She has an MBE for services rendered,' Auntie confided proudly. She had always been impressed by these things.

I was highly sceptical of both claims and was about to say so when I caught sight of the woman spying on us. A long mirror had been placed by the door. 'Matron' was keeping a wary eye on us from the hallway.

I found the whole set-up deeply unsettling.

May Richardson, Auntie's retired maid, who still lived in the house, confirmed some of my fears when I spoke to her about it. She told me that Bob Hutchinson had got Auntie to sign legal documents

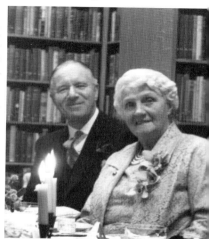

Auntie on her 80th birthday with Bob Hutchinson, her accountant

giving him power of attorney. He could now do whatever he wished with what she owned, acting as if in her name. She had overheard him boasting about certain changes he was to make, not only in the running of the Strangers' Rest Mission, but also in the various companies that came into Auntie's ownership after her husband had died. When he had been asked if he could indeed make those changes, he had replied, 'Why not? I am the major shareholder.'

He now ran the mission. Years earlier he had given up his job to help out at the mission and when Auntie's accountant had retired Bob had taken over – taken over in more senses than one, it seemed.

May told me that 'matron ' was a Mrs Wells, whom Bob had indeed brought in to look after Auntie. May thought Auntie was frightened of her, and she herself did not trust the woman an inch. She had seen Mrs Wells leaving the house with bags of Auntie's silver and other valuables, with Bob's apparent approval. Another thing she felt uneasy about was the fact that Bob ordered cases of sherry and wine in Mrs André's name. Auntie had always been a strict teetotaller – it was part of her Christian convictions.

It was not long before I was in London again. This time I rang Bob Hutchinson. I wanted to see Auntie. He was rather cagey.

'Auntie's been a little poorly,' he said. 'She's not able to see anybody for a week or two.'

He had himself long since taken to calling her 'Auntie'.

'But she'll see me, Bob,' I protested. 'Of course she will!'

He arranged to pick me up at the hospital the next day. When he arrived I noticed he was driving Auntie's car. First, despite my protestations, he took me for lunch at a restaurant in Tottenham Court Road. There he eventually confided that Auntie had suffered a mild heart attack and it would not be wise to put too much strain on her at present.

'I should think it's frustration,' I said. 'Apoplexy from being looked after by that woman.'

'Do you mean Mrs Wells? She's a first rate nurse. She was a matron, you know, and a she's an MBE – '

'Yes, for services rendered,' I interrupted. 'I know. That's what you told Auntie. She was very impressed. Anyway, I should like to pay her a visit, please. And you know, I can always look after her. I promised Auntie, years ago, that I would if she ever became ill.'

'Oh, come, Mina. You can't do that. Not with your career and your family to think of.'

'I would come tomorrow if she asked me,' I replied.

We left the restaurant and got into the car. I imagined Bob had relented and was taking me to see Auntie. It was not long before I realised we were heading in the wrong direction. We were on Commercial Road in the East End.

'This isn't the way to Cheam,' I protested.

'No, Mina. I told you, Auntie can't see you today. I'm taking you to see the mission rooms. You'll be interested in the improvement we've made.'

We stopped at some traffic lights. I felt like getting out there and then. But I didn't. I kept my counsel. And Bob showed me round his mission.

'You know, I have to be careful with Mrs Wells, he said as we walked round the building. 'She's a good nurse for Auntie, and I don't want to lose her. She might be upset if you suddenly turned up again, in view of her explicit advice to the contrary.'

'What's she got to be frightened of?' I said. 'That's what I'd like to know.'

I saw Auntie once more before she died. I had Douglas and David with me and she was at pains to point out an antique oak corner cupboard full of china.

'I should like you to have that, Mina,' she said. 'I'll make sure it's yours.'

She seemed so much older and more frail since the last time I had seen her. The rooms appeared emptier now, too. Many beautiful pieces of furniture, valuable ornaments and familiar trinkets had simply disappeared.

'Auntie, where's that lovely colour photograph of you that was on the mantelpiece?' If she was to give me anything to remember her by, that would have been my choice.

She gave it a moment's thought then said, 'Oh, Bob's brother took that. He said it was a nice picture of me, and just slipped it into his jacket. "You won't be wanting that, will you, Auntie?" he said. I didn't like to argue. It did have a very nice frame. I would have liked you to have that, dearest.'

'Oh, Auntie,' I said. It was almost more than I could bear. But there seemed to be nothing I could do. I was so sad for her.

Not long after, I received a letter from Bertram Craig, her solicitors, informing me of the death of Mrs André. It was the first I had heard of it. The shock came like a body blow – though I suppose I should have been expecting it. The letter listed the many beneficiaries of her will. Bob Hutchinson was the major beneficiary. Most of the rest were relations of his. Bob's brother was to receive £250. I was to receive the same. There was no mention of the oak cupboard. I had not even been invited to the funeral.

I thought back to the time in Sweden, and the other occasions, when Auntie had said, 'One day, Mina, your boat will come in.' We had seemed so close then. She had been more than an adopted aunt. More like a real mother. I felt the loss keenly, and confess I had some bitter thoughts about Bob Hutchinson, and the way – so it had seemed to me – he had blatantly manipulated Auntie to serve his own ends.

It was a struggle for me to let go of the bitterness I felt, but in the end I gave it up to the Lord, who says in Deuteronomy: 'To me belongeth vengeance, and recompense.'

I was still happily working at the Hull School of Nursing when I celebrated my sixtieth birthday. It was March 1968.

I said nothing about it to anybody at work. I did not feel my age, so did not see why I should talk about it. Douglas felt the same about his age. In fact, not even David knew what our real ages were. At least, that had been the case when he was much younger. A teacher had once been amused to tell us that when she had gone round the class getting the boys and girls to say how old their fathers were, David had seemed absolutely to believe that his father was one hundred and twenty-seven years old! This was because we used to joke about our ages whenever David asked us. I would normally say something like 'Over twenty one' or 'As old as my tongue and a little bit older than my teeth'. On that occasion Douglas had said he was one hundred and twenty-seven. David, who must have been about six at the time, had believed it. He only told the class what he thought was correct.

Anyway, the day of my sixtieth birthday came and went. A few weeks later I received a message from the matron – now Miss Morgan Grey. She would like to see me. Would I call at her office? I went along.

'Mrs Banks, I understand that you are sixty years of age.'

'Yes,' I said. 'As it happens, I am. What does that matter?'

'We had a committee meeting yesterday,' she went on, 'and it happened to come up. We all felt so foolish because we knew nothing about it.'

'I don't feel sixty, so why should I talk about it? I don't feel it at all.'

'Well, you know, in the hospital it's a time of retirement. You're supposed to retire at sixty.'

'I don't see why I should. I can still work. I've been working hard, right up until now. I can go on working for a good few years yet.'

'Well now, we'll have to see about that. But I was told that I must bring the matter to your attention.'

'Right you are, matron. Thank you,' I said, and we left it at that.

The next day the financial officer came to see me. 'It was a great shock to all of us to hear that you were sixty,' he said. 'We knew nothing about it.'

'As I said to matron , if I don't feel sixty, why should I broadcast it?'

'Well, I'm telling you now for your own good, nobody can actually make you retire. You may stay in your present position for another five years. If you want to retire in that time, you can do so. Go any time you like, Mrs Banks. But remember, nobody can force you. It's entirely up to you.'

I didn't need to think about it. 'I'd rather stay,' I told him at once. 'I enjoy my work and I'll continue to do it, if I may.'

'That's perfectly acceptable,' he said. Then, with a twinkle in his eye, he added, 'You'll continue to be paid, of course. Good luck.'

As soon as David reached the age of seventeen he started taking driving lessons, and when he passed his test – the first time! – he also began to use the car. Actually, it ended up with his taking me to school and dropping me off, before going on to the grammar school. Between us we clocked up thousands of miles. The mileometer would soon be doing a complete cycle and returning to zero. My little car was losing some of its zippiness and in first gear and reverse it made a loud clanking noise.

'You know, I think you'll need a new engine soon,' Douglas said one day.

'Is that an expensive business?' I asked.

'Well, it'll be about eighty or ninety pounds.'

'Oh, dear,' I said, 'I don't know if I'll be able to afford that.'

David had overheard our conversation. After a while, he said, 'If I save up the money and buy the engine, would you let me have the car?'

'But you'll never be able to get that much money,' I said.

'Yes, I will. I've got money in the Halifax. That'll go towards it.'

When David was born, Douglas's friend Harold Brocklebank had opened a Halifax Building Society savings account for David and put £5 in to start it off. From that time on, we put any gifts of money for him in the account. He saved money of his own too, so that by now he had about £70 altogether. He had won a place at Manchester University and had been thinking of buying a motor scooter or motorbike, but Douglas and I much preferred that he have the car. Douglas had retired by this time, so it would be easier now for us to share our other car.

David did save. In the summer holidays between school and university I was able to get him a job as a porter at the hospital. His first week's wages of £16 was stolen as he was taking a shower after work one day, but he didn't let that dishearten him, and when he had enough to pay for the engine, Geoff Skin, a mechanic friend of ours – the husband of one of my old student nurses – replaced it for him. I had said he could have the car if he saved up and had the engine replaced. He had done just that, so now Ebenezer was his.

He and his girlfriend Annabelle took to calling it Ulysses. He learned about maintaining the car, and filled and painted the areas of rust, and really took good care of it. The car that Eddie drove served us all magnificently. David had it for another eight years until the replacement engine had worn out and the speedometer had returned to zero once again. And even then, when Ebenezer would go no faster than twenty miles an hour and there was more rust and plastic padding than metal in its bodywork, he was able to sell it on – for its unusual number plate: 50 MPJ.

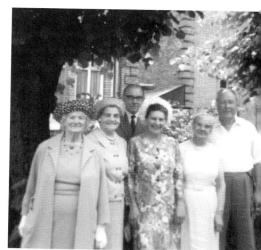

Last gathering of the four sisters with Douglas and
Frank outside Number Five Eldon Grove, 1969

15

Trip of a Lifetime

…if you can gain your freedom, avail yourself of the opportunity!
1 Corinthians 7.21

In 1972 Douglas and I went on a trip to Canada and America. Mr Bates, Chairman of the Hull 'A' Group Hospital Committee, who had been so kind at the time of my appointment as deputy principal, was instrumental in bringing it about.

'Wouldn't you like a sabbatical?' he asked me one day.

'Yes, I would,' I replied. 'Douglas and I have often talked about taking a cruise to Canada. I have a sister and cousins there, and Douglas lived over there when he was a little boy. We'd love to do that. Perhaps see something of America too.'

'How long would you need?' he asked.

'Well, it would take us four or five weeks to sail there and the same to get back. I suppose we would need about…' I did a quick calculation, '…four months?' I suggested, none too hopefully.

'Take it,' he said.

I wrote to Miss Lambert, the matron, explaining that Mr Bates was encouraging me to have a four-month sabbatical and that I wished to take up his suggestion. Replying, she acknowledged that if Mr Bates was behind the idea then I had the right to take leave if I wished. But she added, 'I'm afraid I don't agree with the taking of sabbaticals. Once people in your position start taking them, any Tom, Dick and Harry will be asking. It's not good for the running of the hospital.'

Douglas found her attitude most upsetting. 'After all you've done for them over the last twenty years,' he complained when I showed him the letter. But I didn't allow myself to get worked up about it. As long as I could go.

In any case, the trip was partly in connection with my hospital work. I already had long-standing invitations to three Canadian hospitals, and while I was over there I intended to visit other hospitals as the opportunity presented itself, to see how their practice and teaching compared to ours. We had every excuse to travel widely, for there were many friends and relations who were eager to offer us hospitality, and for the same reason accommodation would pose no problem. And added to the personal and professional aspects of our adventure, there was a third strand: as President of the Hull branch of the international club of professional women called the Soroptimists, I was requested to make contact with various branches throughout Canada, and extend the hand of friendship as a representative of the British Soroptimists.

When I was outlining my plans to Mr Bates, he immediately saw the professional potential. 'When you visit these hospitals,' he said, 'perhaps you would note anything that might be of help to us here and then get something down on paper when you get back.'

This I readily agreed to do, and on our return I put together a comprehensive report which I hope made some contribution to the Health Authority's plans for its future development.

I also wrote an account for our friends to read. I called it *The Trip of a Lifetime*.

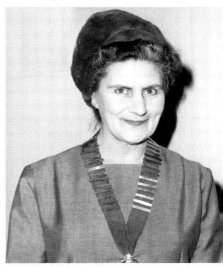

President of Hull Soroptimists, 1969

I had told Mr Bates that we hoped to travel to Canada by ship. When we got down to making specific arrangements, we found there were no British ships sailing that route, so the travel agency booked us on a Polish ship going out and a Russian ship for our return.

We left Tilbury docks under a grey sky. But once the white cliffs of Dover had passed from sight, we had three days of uninterrupted sunshine which we spent relaxing on the sun deck. Three days of mist and cold followed, then two very rough days – but nothing like the experience of our honeymoon trip to Jersey those twenty years earlier! Approaching Newfoundland, we spotted a number of icebergs in the distance. The weather became warmer again and it was under a brilliant blue sky that we entered the Gulf of St Lawrence.

The temperature was a humid 99° as we disembarked at the immense harbour of Old Montreal, overlooked by its magnificent Church of Notre Dame. The next day we made our way to Brantford by train and were met by my dear sister Jean. We stayed with her for a week before setting off on our further travels, making a lightning trip through America on the network of 'Greyhound' coaches, stopping first at Detroit, where on a tour of Ford's factory we witnessed the complete assembly of a car in seventy minutes – though the experience was not an encouragement to own such a car! But Henry Ford was not only interested in cars. He was also the founder of the now world-famous Ford Hospital and its Clara Ford Nurses School and Residence. A visit to this hospital was the first of my professional engagements on the trip.

We left Detroit early one morning to continue our journey across the States from East to West, passing through Chicago, Denver and finally arriving at California and the huge sprawling city of Los Angeles, where we were introduced to one of the rarer delicacies of the American diet which had not yet made its way to the UK – Kentucky Fried Chicken. It was unnerving to see on every corner the large advertising hoardings with the genial face of its inventor,

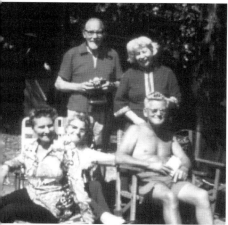

At Long Point, Ontario, with Jean and friends

Colonel Saunders, with his white goatee beard, smiling down on us. Unnerving, because he bore an uncanny resemblance to Douglas, who had recently been cultivating a white goatee beard of his own. We had been wondering why people were giving us strange looks…

The Reverend Doctor Phillip Ray and his wife Peggy were our hosts and we stayed with them for several days in their beautiful Long Beach home. The Christian fellowship was sweet and with them we visited many places, ranging from the ridiculous to the sublime, including Disneyland – 'The Happiest Place On Earth' – and the San Juan Capistrano Mission in San Diego, where on St Joseph's day thousands of swallows fly in from the Pacific to build their nests in the ruins of the chapel.

Returning to Canada via the states of Oregon and Washington, we found we were in a land of breathtaking beauty: lakes, mountains, forests and waterfalls. As we left the USA, going through Customs at Seattle and entering the Canadian State of British Columbia, there was a noticeable change: miles upon miles of recently planted forests of spruce and fir, with the occasional clearing for a logging station to load up its lumber wagons.

In Vancouver we met up once again with my sister and a cousin. Indeed, throughout the whole trip I discovered cousins I'd no idea I had. They and their friends gave us a splendid welcome wherever we went and they were always delighted to hear of news from the Old Country.

From Vancouver we travelled through heavy rain towards the town of Banff and the Canadian Rockies. As we drove into the mountains the grey mists lifted, the sun broke through and a rainbow arched across the mountains. In Banff itself we watched a spectacular parade of Mounties and tribal Indians in the main street, and I spotted a notice in a drugstore for visiting Soroptimists to contact the local group. I rang the number given, and the evening was spent in the delightful company of two of the local members: true Soroptimism.

One of the most memorable days of the entire trip was when Douglas was able to visit his childhood home town of Peterborough, just the other side of Toronto. He had been taken to live there by his parents when he was about ten years of age. He still had the piece torn from the local paper which carried the announcement of their arrival to settle in the country. As it turned out, after barely more than a year in the place, his father – who could never stay in one place for long – decided it was time for the family to return to England. But that brief period in Canada had made an indelible impression on Douglas, and though Peterborough had changed considerably he was fascinated to recognise certain landmarks. Amazingly, we found that his old school was still standing, and he was able to sit in his old classroom – possibly even at the same desk!

We watched a game of baseball and talked to local inhabitants about the various changes which had come about in the sixty years that Douglas had been away. Then we lunched at a picnic site alongside the waterway where the Peterborough 'Lift Lock', a masterpiece of engineering, allowed ships and boats to pass from one water basin to another. Later we walked along the banks of the Trent river, back into town, and in the early evening returned by coach to Brantford. We calculated that we had walked over twenty miles that day.

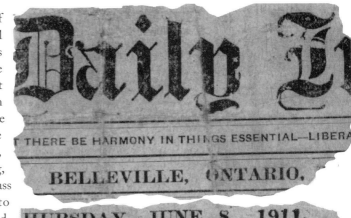

All the days we spent in Canada were packed with things to do and see as our tour took in Calgary, Edmonton, the Niagara Falls, Scarborough, on the edge of Lake Ontario, and Ottawa, where we were guided around the beautiful Parliament buildings. We climbed the Peace Tower and looked down upon Hull, Ontario, and were reminded of Hull, England. We went into the mountains to the Vermilion Lakes where part of Doctor Zhivago was filmed. We were guests at several Soroptimist functions: in Montreal I was introduced to the Nursing Superintendent of the St John's Ambulance Brigade who took us round the sites of the Old Town; in Alberta the Soroptimist President, Professor of the University Nursing Faculty, invited us for dinner in the revolving restaurant tower of Chateau Lacombe – as we ate, so we watched the city move below us as darkness fell and the lights of the city sprang into life. As for material for my report, in the end we were welcomed at a total of nineteen hospitals and schools of nursing.

The return voyage was on the Russian ship *Alexander Pushkin*. The entertainment on board was excellent. We attended Russian language classes and joined in the dancing classes, and received a diploma for 'surviving' both. Not so good was the food, which was for the most part tasteless. An added difficulty was that our baggage had been placed in an inaccessible part of the hold, so we had to make do with a weekend case of clothes for the whole ten-day voyage. But these shortcomings were more than compensated for by the classical concerts and lively discussions with new-found friends.

We disembarked at Tilbury – to be greeted by dock strikes, grey drizzle and dirty trains. We were home.

In the afterglow of our trip, it seemed that life could never be quite the same again. But inevitably after a few months back at work, the vivid splendour and excitement of it all receded as we settled back into our normal routine. We still had our memories of it though. And what wonderful memories they were.

One day, out of the blue, Mr Reeve asked me what I would like as a present.

'A present. Why?' I said.

'For your retirement. We all get a present on retirement.'

It was 1973. I was sixty-five and retirement could not be put off any longer.

'Oh, I don't know,' I said. 'It hadn't occurred to me I'd be getting a retirement present.'

'Well, think over what you want, and let me know.'

I gave it some thought. It would be useful to have a slide projector. We had taken a lot of slides on our trip to Canada and the USA. 'Would that be all right?' I asked Mr Reeve when I saw him next. 'A slide projector and perhaps a screen.'

'Yes, I think we can probably manage that.'

A couple of days later Jane Humber phoned me. She was a journalist with the *Hull Daily Mail* who had a regular column on Thursday nights. 'I wondered if I could come and interview you, Mrs Banks. The hospital has been in touch with our paper and said you have had a long and interesting career in nursing.'

When she came round she asked me about my training and previous work, my qualifications, what I had done and where I'd been. One of the things which interested her was my time in Malta.

The next Thursday a copy of the *Hull Daily Mail* was sent to me, and there it all was. It spoke of Malta and other things, and my impending retirement. The article caused quite a stir in the hospital – not least because they had no idea I was about to retire.

There was no chance to slow down. I was working hard right up to the last day, though it was punctuated by farewell treats. The day before I was to leave for good, the nurses in my class wanted me to have lunch with them in a nearby pub called The Anchor. At the end of my last morning, Mr Reeve brought out a bottle of sherry and a packet of nuts, which the school staff shared in my office.

'Come along,' he said, 'Sister Morris and I are taking you out for a bar lunch.' We had steak sandwiches and a shandy. It was very nice. When we got back I had to pack. During the afternoon Douglas arrived to help me with my things.

At the end of the day there was an official retirement party. The catering staff had put on a lovely tea and Mrs Brocklebank, the new chairman of the hospital committee, presented me with the slide projector and screen, and gave a little speech. Mr Reeve said a few words, and then various nurses and colleagues came up with more retirement gifts. One parcel turned out to be a case to hold all my slides in. Another was a plant in a beautiful pot. 'It isn't the plant, sister, so much as the pot,' said the nurse. 'It's been specially made.'

'Thank you,' I said.

When it was all over, Douglas was there to help carry my things to the car.

I felt extremely sad about retiring. But I thought, oh well, I'll look upon it as a holiday at first, and not having any responsibilities will be rather lovely. So that's what I did.

There was the opportunity to see to things at home which needed doing. Douglas and I decorated throughout Number Five, clambering up ladders to hang wallpaper in the high-

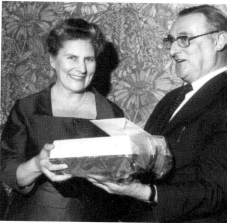

The retirement presentation, 1973

ceilinged rooms, making the flats and bedsitting rooms we had created more comfortable for their occupants. It was a joy to be able to spend more time with Douglas. He was always so loving and interested in everything I did. He stood by me and was a great help in many ways.

There was also more time for the various organisations with which I had become involved over the years. I took on the position of General Secretary to the Ladies' Musical Union. It meant a lot of extra work but I enjoyed it very much.

We would have practice sessions every Monday night in a church hall opposite Park Street and gave concerts four times a year. Only women were allowed to be members of the choir and come to the concerts, and we had female guest artists. But once a year we had what was called the Gentlemen's Evening, to which husbands, brothers, fathers and sons were all invited, and the concert would include male as well as female guest artists.

The concert would be held at the Guildhall with a meal afterwards in the Banqueting Room, whose walls were lined with paintings of Kingston upon Hull through the ages as it developed from the little village of Wyke, owned by the monks at Beverley in medieval times, through the bustling port and fish-marketing town which became a city by king's decree, through the devastation of the war years, to the modern metropolis it was fast becoming, known for its shopping centres, thriving university and Humber Bridge, which after years of planning was finally about to be built.

Around that time I was also elected to the Hull Health Council Committee. We met regularly at 83 Ferensway – general meetings on Thursdays and study groups on Mondays. The task of my study group was to visit hospitals and nursing homes, talking with patients and staff to assess the effectiveness of the Area Health Service provision, to listen to any complaints and consider suggestions for improvements. Long waiting lists were always a cause of complaint.

Our views were canvassed concerning the fluoridation of water. I felt strongly about it. In my paper to the Council I said it was wrong for fluoride to be put into our drinking water. Why should we be forced to drink fluoridated water when we knew that too great a concentration of fluoride caused bone tumours? Would it not be better if fluoride was made available in tablet form? Those who wanted it could then take measured doses of fluoride, rather as they might take a vitamin pill.

My paper was copied and distributed to the rest of the committee, and when we went to Harrogate for a major conference on the subject I had to stand up and outline the reasons I felt so strongly about it. It was a contravention of basic human rights, I explained, that everybody should be forced to drink water containing fluoride. It left no room for individual choice.

My work for the General Nursing Council continued, and took up an increasing part of my time. I went to most hospitals in the UK to adjudicate at the written examinations and to supervise the practical examinations. There were piles of exam papers to mark and assess, in collaboration with the doctors and specialists who were my co-examiners. All expenses were paid on top of the examining fee. Now that I no longer had my little car, I opted to travel by train. Happily, the Council ensured their examiners travelled first class, which was quite a novelty and most relaxing. All in all, I felt that my nursing and teaching experience was being put to good use, even in retirement.

There was more time now for seeing friends and socialising. Douglas and I made trips all over the country, looking up old friends, going to see David – who was now a graduate in drama and had taken a postgraduate diploma at the Bristol Old Vic Theatre School. He was working as an actor in theatres far and wide, and we tried to catch his performances when we could.

We became close friends with one of the young people who was staying in the downstairs bedsit that David had been using as a study before he went to university. She was a lovely Chinese girl called Mo Wah Leong. But she was known to us as Viva. She was a Christian and a dietician at the Hull Royal Infirmary. Since she was a long way from her home in Hong Kong and her parents were not Christians, she took to calling us her 'God-mum' and 'God-dad'. So, of course, we thought of her as our spiritual daughter. It seemed so fortuitous that she had come to us. I had wanted a daughter as well as a son. Now here was Viva. And I had so wanted to go to China. Now, I thought, the Lord has brought China to me.

Viva took up training at the All Nations' Bible College and became a missionary, working among the Chinese communities in Britain. She has remained a life-long and much-loved friend.

I was still President of the Hull Soroptimists. Retirement had given me more time to devote to my activities there. The name Soroptimist – deriving from the Latin for sister, *soror*, and the word *optimist* – gives a good idea of its guiding principle: to encourage women, internationally, to be the best of sisters to each other. The Objects of Soroptimism in full are stated thus:

> To maintain high ethical standards in business, the professions and other aspects of life. To strive for human rights for all people and, in particular, to

advance the status of women. To develop a spirit of friendship and unity amongst Soroptimists of all countries. To quicken the spirit of service and human understanding. To contribute to international understanding and universal friendship.

The group met on a regular basis and one of our objectives was to raise funds for various charitable events. At one of their fund-raising dinners, shortly after my retirement, I was going from table to table welcoming people and chatting to them. At one table sat Jane Humber, the women's columnist from the *Hull Daily Mail* who had interviewed me before my retirement. Her real name was Barbara Robinson. Sitting beside her was her husband, Peter. She introduced me to him.

'I was very interested in Jane's piece on you in the paper,' he said. ' Your experiences in Malta and so forth.'

'Oh, yes?'

'Yes, indeed,' he went on. 'You ought to write a book.'

'A book? I couldn't write a book. Good gracious!'

'Peter's absolutely right,' said Barbara. 'You just make up your mind to get down to it. That's all it takes.'

It seemed an impossible idea. But their encouragement stuck in my mind. I often thought afterwards how I might make a start one day. The trouble was I always seemed to have so much to do.

But the seed was there. Barbara's interview had given me an opportunity to review something of my life, to recall how wonderfully the Lord had looked after me: all through my training and the various hospitals I had worked for, all through Malta and all the many other things I had done, the places I had seen, the people I had met.

One day, I thought, maybe I will get those memoirs done.

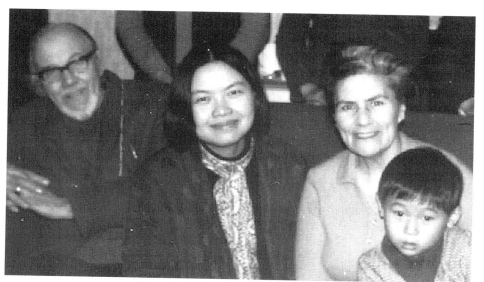

Viva (Mo Wah) Leong, our spiritual daughter

16

Stroke

By your endurance you will gain your lives
Luke 21.19

For many years I had wanted to move out of the centre of Hull. Number Five was a rambling old house, difficult to maintain, and though we had made the best of the large flat we lived in at the top of the house, it was not a place where visitors could easily be accommodated and entertained, and it was a struggle to keep it clean and looking presentable.

Douglas had made all sorts of improvements and modernisations since the first (and last) time Auntie Dagmar had visited us, but I was nevertheless a little ashamed that we were still living there, twenty-five years later.

The houses in Eldon Grove were becoming neglected and increasingly run-down. Too large now to serve as family homes, they were being turned one by one into poorly converted flats. At Number Five, which had once been just two flats, we had a succession of young people – Viva had been one of them, in the early Seventies – living in the four flats or bedsits Douglas had now created. What had originally been Marjorie Beevers' flat was now a smaller flat at the back and two bedsitting rooms. The flat on the first floor, which Douglas had converted from the old Covenantor Room after his retirement, was also occupied.

Between the two of us, we would keep the place decorated and well cared for. The fact that we were now both in our seventies did not stop us getting out the stepladders and roller brushes and toiling late into the night to paint the main hallway – which must have been thirty or so feet high at the stairwell. It kept us active – at least that could be said in favour of owning Number Five. We could also put people up at short notice. A couple of years earlier, when David had unexpectedly got an acting job at the Humberside Theatre in Hull, we had been able to provide him with self-contained accommodation because the first floor flat had become vacant.

But that coincidence of fortune was unlikely to be repeated. He was now going to be living in London with Maureen, an actress he had met the previous year while working at the Welsh National Drama Company. And I was longing to move into some little bungalow on the outskirts of Hull. Something with a pretty garden which would require minimal upkeep, so that I could concentrate on my various interests and activities: I was still an active member of the Soroptimists, the League of Friends, and the Ladies' Musical Union; and President of the Western General Hospital League, Secretary of the Hull College of Nursing and Member-in-Charge of the local St John's Ambulance Brigade.

Nothing was stopping us from making the move. We had saved hard over the years and had managed to put away enough to buy a small place outright. The real stumbling block was that deep down Douglas just did not like the idea of moving. When he was very young his father and mother had moved almost every year. It left him with a desire just to stay put. However, even he was at last coming round to the idea. So at the start of 1977 we began in earnest to look for something that would suit us for the sum of money we had available.

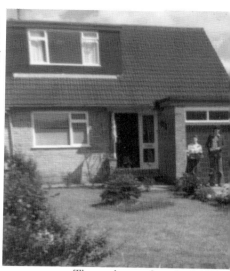

The new house at Swanland, 1977

After months of viewing properties that were never quite right, we came upon the little semi-detached house in Swanland, 86 Mill Rise, that I now think of as home. It was not a bungalow, since it was built on two floors, but with its low roof and dormer windows it had the feel of a bungalow. Swanland was a pretty village about nine miles out of Hull, complete with village pond, a family of swans and lots of ducks. A couple of miles down the road was North Ferriby, which was where Marjorie Beevers had come to live ten or fifteen years earlier. We had always kept in close touch with Marjorie. It was lovely to think that we might be neighbours after all this time.

We paid the £17,000 asking price in cash and moved in during the summer. Wondering what to call it, we thought of the text 'In Him we live and move and have our being' – the text that had brought us together. We felt sure the Lord had brought us here and that he would be with us, so we decided to call our new home *Inhimwe*.

One of the first things Douglas had done was to have a large porch built at the front door to function as a kind of sun-lounge. We put in a couple of small armchairs and a small table and often had tea in there. It was a real suntrap. At the back door, using old bricks and a couple of doors from a demolition site, he built a lean-to for use as a utility room, doing all the work himself. We bought a chest freezer for it, and much later, a tumble-drier. But that was to be after an event which changed our lives suddenly, and forever.

The first hour of every day I spent gardening. I just loved it. I loved the smell of the earth. I loved to see things grow, as I planted them. That first year I grew lettuces and chives. We had enough to feed us throughout the year.

One morning during the August of 1980, Douglas decided he had a lot of shopping to do. I had started gardening and had begun to prune the hedges and trees at the front of the house. He came to the door and shouted, 'We must go shopping, darling. Come on!'

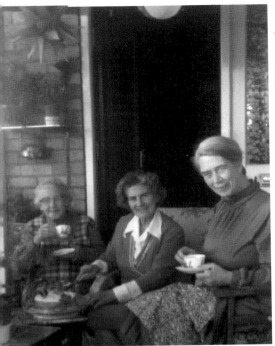

Marjorie Beevers and Kathleen Dennis in the sun-lounge

'All right,' I said. 'I'll finish these when I come back.'

I hurriedly changed from my gardening clothes and off we went in the car to the shops in Anlaby and Hessle.

When we got back, we had a quick lunch and I went out to finish the pruning. I had left my saw hanging on the laburnum tree to mark where I had got to. I grabbed hold of it and started work again. I was stretching up, sawing through one of the thicker laburnum branches when suddenly there was a loud bang.

I thought the branch had broken loose and struck my head. It was the last thought I had before darkness enveloped me. For a long time I knew no more.

I came back to semi-consciousness in hospital three weeks later. I had not been hit by a falling branch. The bang had been a blood vessel rupturing in my head. I had suffered a particularly severe cerebral haemorrhage, or stroke.

For a long time I had no memory of the events leading up to the stroke, and I still have little recollection of what happened immediately afterwards, though it appears I did remain partly conscious for about half an hour. Douglas was to tell me – much later, when I could take it in – that he had heard my raised voice in the garden. He thought I was talking to a neighbour or a visitor. He came to the front door to see who it was, but I was nowhere to be seen. The car was in the driveway, and suddenly he caught sight of me, on my hands and knees, crawling round the side of it, calling 'Douglas! Douglas!'

He didn't know what had happened or what he should do, but he came to me and somehow – he didn't know how he managed it – dragged me over the porch step and on to one of the armchairs. Apparently I was conscious enough to say, 'Ring Marjorie, she'll know what to do.' So he rang Marjorie Beevers. A neighbour brought her up to Swanland immediately.

'We must get the doctor,' she said to Douglas as soon as she saw me.

Our own doctor was not on duty that day, so the surgery sent a locum. I was more or less in coma when he arrived, but I came round enough to realise he was a stranger.

'Who are you?' I asked.

'I'm a doctor, Mrs Banks,' he said. 'I've come because your doctor's away. I'm here to help you.'

Marjorie said he was marvellous with me. He examined me thoroughly, and then he arranged for me to go to Beverley Westwood Hospital.

My next vivid memory is of the Christmas trees on the ward. My bed was close to one of them. Four months had passed since that day I had been pruning the laburnum. In that time a lot had happened of which I have only vague recollections. David, Douglas and Marjorie gave me a full account of it.

David came up to Hull immediately Marjorie phoned him to tell him what had happened. Maureen came with him. She was working at the Connaught Theatre in Worthing, but it was August bank holiday and she was able to get away. When she left, to get back in time for the Tuesday evening performance, things were still looking pretty bad for me.

During the weeks that followed, Douglas, David and Marjorie continued to visit the hospital twice and sometimes three times a day. The doctor told them to expect the worst. The longer a stroke victim remains unconscious, he warned them, the less chance there is of survival.

'I'm sorry,' he said. 'There's very little more we can do. Even if she does regain consciousness she will probably be severely brain-damaged. Or she will contract a chest infection and she'll not be strong enough to shake it off.'

Marjorie took a fatalistic view. She was soon organising David to get our address book up to date and wanted to place an order for black-edged cards with the printers in preparation for the inevitable. But there were plenty of other things for David to do, helping his father with the many things that had to be seen to. In a way, they were relieved to be occupied with something else.

One of the first things David did was to take his father into town and buy an automatic washing machine and that tumble-drier. Before my stroke I had been using an old twin-tub. We used to hang the wet clothes on a rotary drying line in the garden and watch out for the rain. David realised that if I survived, everyday routines like washing clothes would have to be made as easy as possible. When the washer arrived, Douglas said, 'We must get a plumber.'

'No,' said David, 'I'll do it.'

He bought the necessary equipment from the local DIY store. Douglas told me he was expecting a flood as David worked, cutting and connecting all the various pipes and tubes, but no, he did it perfectly. That washing-machine has been such a blessing throughout the years, and even now, fifteen years later, it is still going strong.

They decided to put Number Five up for sale. It was our third year at *Inhimwe*, but we were still struggling to maintain the old house and see to the tenants. I had been unable to get Douglas finally to have done with the place. It was full of old bits and pieces which he was reluctant to get rid of – ancient vacuum cleaners and electric fires, heavy wooden trestle tables salvaged from the camps at Ulrome, bits of the old motorcycle he used to have when I first knew him, and David's rusting pushbike which Douglas was determined to repair – and yet it would have been impossible to have all these things at our little house in Swanland.

David saw that Douglas must be free of this additional burden. He persuaded his father that Number Five should be sold. Between them, they cleared it of the remaining possessions, gave notice to the tenants, and put it into the hands of an estate agent. Marianne Tansey and my godson, her son Christopher, were a great help at this time. They transported seven carloads of junk to the local jumble sale.

Friends helped in any way they could. Ken and Grace Gibbs, as ever, were a great support. A newer friend, Dr Peter Nelson, a chemistry lecturer at the university and active member of Trafalgar Street Church, provided much needed spiritual and emotional support, and has done so unfailingly ever since.

With bereavements and accidents the survivors often blame themselves for what has happened. It was like this with Douglas. He felt the clutter in his life had become a burden on me and weighed me down. Fervently, day after day, Douglas prayed, 'Bring her back to me, Lord. Give me just one more chance.'

One of my earliest recollections after my stroke was of Douglas kneeling beside my hospital bed, tears streaming down his face. 'Oh, darling,' he said, 'the Lord's given you back to me. I promise it will never happen again.'

'It wasn't your fault,' I said.

'Yes, it was. I allowed you to do too much.'

I had been leading a busy life. The Soroptimists, the League of Friends, the Ladies' Musical Union, St John's Ambulance Brigade – I had each of their different meetings to attend. I was also doing some part-time teaching at the College of Technology. But I had chosen to do those things, and enjoyed them. Douglas had no reason to blame himself. But he did. I think that is why he agreed to sell Number Five and get rid of so many things he had previously wanted to hang on to. He thought they had placed an added strain on our lives and felt, rightly or wrongly, that they had contributed to my stroke. It was something he could do for me, if only the Lord would bring me back to him.

David had been in touch by letter or by phone with all our friends to let them know what had happened. One of them was Kathleen Dennis, a colleague and dear friend from my time at the Western General School. When we were working together twenty years before, she herself had suffered a stroke. She had been in her early fifties and she made a complete recovery.

As David described my condition, she became anxious to tell him what had happened to her while she was still in coma. What she had to say was this. A friend had stayed by her bed and spoken her name and kept talking to her, despite the fact that she appeared to be deeply unconscious. Kathleen was convinced that by doing this her friend had saved her, for she was aware of her friend's voice, and wanted so much to respond. One day the friend was talking to her and holding her hand. She said, 'If you can hear me, Kathleen, squeeze my hand.' Kathleen concentrated on squeezing her friend's hand, and her friend felt a movement in Kathleen's fingers. It was faint, but it was certainly there. The friend continued to encourage Kathleen to squeeze her hand. Over the next few days, the responses grew stronger. And then at last Kathleen emerged from the coma.

'Try it with your mother,' Kathleen urged David. 'You must talk to her as if she can hear you.'

So after that, whenever they came to see me, David and Douglas held my hand and talked to me. David would say, 'Mother, if you can hear me, squeeze my hand.' But they felt no response.

The hospital was eight miles from Swanland. Douglas and David continued to visit me regularly. Marjorie came along almost as often. They sometimes brought a packed lunch, and after they left me they would go to the Westwood, have a picnic under the trees, then come back in the afternoon.

Marjorie was now eighty-six years old. From time to time, Douglas would suggest she stayed at home, afraid that she might be taking on too much. But she was alert and very strong-minded, and this only made her more resolute. She had once promised to look after Douglas if anything should happen to me and she was determined to keep to her word. The secret of her vitality, she believed, was in the nap she always took after lunch. She encouraged Douglas to do the same.

The visits continued. I had tubes everywhere, Douglas said. I was being fed intragastrically through a Ryles tube which was passed into the nostril and down the back of the throat and oesophagus and into my stomach. I was catheterised, of course, and I also had a drip tube inserted into a vein on the back of my hand. I was losing weight and must have looked a pathetic sight. Douglas and David continued to hold my hand and talk to me. There was still no response. On the contrary, I seemed to be sinking further away from them. They were both terribly upset.

The next day I seemed a little more stable. David was holding my hand and talking to me as usual, speaking my name and asking me to squeeze his hand to show that I could hear him. Suddenly, he felt my fingers move against his. It was a slight movement, almost imperceptible. I was showing no other signs of consciousness. He thought he might be imagining it.

The next time they came, the nurse greeted them with a smile. 'There was some improvement in the night,' she said, and they were astonished to see that I was propped a little higher in the bed, still hardly conscious but able to respond a little to their words of greeting. Marjorie had never tried speaking to me when I was unconscious, but now she urged David to say something.

'Tell her what the weather's like,' she suggested.

'It's cold and nasty outside,' said David, holding my hand again.

Apparently, I grimaced.

When they were about to leave, the nurse said to Douglas, 'Doctor wants to see you, Mr Banks.'

'I don't know what's happened,' the doctor said when they went in to see him, 'but your wife seems to be over the worst. As you know, I'd given up hope. But in this sort of circumstance I am always glad to say that I was wrong in my prognosis. I said she would never recover, but she's turned the corner.'

'It's an answer to prayer,' said Marjorie.

Indeed, many people had been praying. Douglas had received letters from relatives and friends scattered all over the world to say that they and their churches were praying for me. My own church, Trafalgar Street, had been mentioning me in their prayer meetings since word of my stroke had reached them. I truly feel I owe my recovery to the Lord: He really does answer prayer.

The improvement continued. A day or two later, a nurse rang from the hospital. 'Oh, Mr Banks, I've encouraging news. Your wife's sitting up, writing.'

The next time they visited, I was being nursed in a fully upright position. The nurse told them she had been marking her charts and she had put her pen and her notepad by my bed. There was also a newspaper lying there. I picked up the pen and started writing my name, Douglas's name and David's name, all round the margins of the paper. The nurse was amazed when she saw it. She gave the page to Douglas when he arrived. He kept and treasured it.

The haemorrhage had been on the right side of the brain. It had left me with hemiplegia – one-sided paralysis. Each side of the brain controls the opposite side of the body. I could move neither my left arm nor left leg. The muscles on the left half of my face were frozen, giving me a lop-sided expression, and there was no sensation down the whole of my left side. In addition, my left field of vision was gone. I had some initial difficulty in learning to speak again, but fortunately this was not long-lasting. Total loss of speech is more common with left-brain haemorrhages.

I was informed that a speech therapist would be coming to see me, to help with my initial speech difficulties. I remembered my elocution lessons with Amman Jones and thought, oh, I'll be prepared for her. When she arrived, I greeted her with the words, somewhat mangled, 'How now brown cow.'

She laughed and said, 'Well, now, has someone been here before me?'

'The rain in Spain is mainly on the plain,' I slurred.

She was not at all put out by my behaviour. Stroke victims often act a little strangely. 'Say stewed prunes and custard,' she instructed.

'Stewed prunes and custard,' I said.

'Fried eggs and bacon?'

'Fried eggs and bacon,' I repeated, my mouth beginning to water. Then I tried one on her. 'King Cophetua and the beggar maid,' I attempted strenuously. 'Do you know that one?'

'No, Mrs Banks, but it's one to remember. Tell you what. Just for now, stick to the ones I gave you. Stewed prunes and custard, and fried eggs and bacon. The doctor will want to hear them when he does his rounds.'

He deserves more than stewed prunes and custard, I thought, but did as I was told.

'Good morning, Mrs Banks,' said the doctor when he came to my bed.

'Stewed prunes and custard,' I annunciated carefully.

He took my hand and patted it. 'That's a good girl,' he said.

My voice was really quite weak because I did not yet have the strength back in my lungs, but later when Douglas, David and Marjorie came to see me, I was able to speak with them a little more easily. Quietly, I said to Douglas, 'I wonder why God has allowed this to come to us?'

'Don't worry, darling,' he said. 'We'll know one day.'

David stayed until it was clear that I was out of danger. Then he went back to London to catch up with his life there. He had managed to be with Douglas for five weeks in all, and in the months – and years – that followed he continued to make extended visits to make sure that Douglas and I were coping with our changed circumstances.

Some months into the next year, it was felt that Douglas could look after me at home. Because I could do very little for myself, he would have to see to my every need. Initially, I went home for a trial fortnight, to see if Douglas would be able to cope.

I was unable to walk, so I could no longer use the stairs. The guest bedroom downstairs was converted for my use. Douglas had the built-in wardrobe taken out and a shower cubicle fitted in its place. Fortunately, just across the hallway from the bedroom and the living room was a small toilet. Douglas found he could lift me from my armchair or my bed, swivel me into the wheelchair, and wheel me to the rather confined space of the toilet.

The nurses at the hospital were trained to look after patients like me, but Douglas wasn't a trained nurse. He had never had any experience of looking after a stroke victim. And he was nearly seventy-nine years old. All he had was his love for me, his strength – he was still physically strong for his age – and his determination. He did find it terribly difficult at first, but oh, how kind he was.

One day he said to me, 'Do you remember, darling, when you were in the hospital you said you wondered why the Lord allowed this to happen? Well, it's brought us closer to Him, and closer to others. Closer to each other, too. I never knew how we would be able to face it, but we did it. The Lord brought us a blessing out of that awful thing. He helped to pull you through.'

Time went on. To give Douglas a break I would go into Kingston General Hospital for a fortnight's respite care every couple of months. One day when David was home for a week, he and Douglas made their usual visit to see me. Marjorie had been ill with a tummy bug and I asked after her.

David broke the news that she had died the previous night. It came as a complete shock. Dear, faithful Marjorie, who had been such a tower of strength when I was so ill, who indeed had been responsible, in some ways, for bringing Douglas and I together, thirty years before.

She had been such a good friend and Christian companion to both of us. She had been quite fond of Douglas before I had come along. It was thought by some at the time that she had an idea of marrying him herself. But if this was so, she never made

Jane Humber Hull Daily Mail July 1981

New president

MRS WINIFRED HARDING has accepted the presidency of North Humberside Centre of the Royal College of Nursing.

She succeeds Mrs Mina Banks, who is now recovering slowly but surely from a serious illness.

Mrs Banks has guided the Centre through a number of important changes, attempting to keep its activities in line with the needs of the membership, and her personal gracious style has been greatly respected.

Sending her a gift of flowers, Centre Chairman Mr T. Morrell wrote: "I do hope that nursing serves you now, in your hour of need, as well as you have served nursing, and we all look forward to hearing much better news of progress and recovery."

And that goes for all of us who know Mina, both in and out of the nursing service.

her feelings known, and never expressed any kind of jealousy towards me. And Douglas had told me he had never felt that way about her.

She had never married, and she left no relatives. But she did have a love for children. She had certainly been good to David, taking a real interest in him, and as 'Auntie' Marjorie – along with 'Granny' Joelson – providing him with the extended family he would not otherwise have had when he was growing up. I had often wondered if she regretted not having any children of her own.

Among her papers was a poem she had written, which may partly answer the question. It was entitled *Treasures Missed:*

> You meet her nearly every morning with her cheery word and smile
> And you think she has no sorrows, that her life is all worth while.
> Have you seen her in the quiet of her little room at night?
> A shadow darkening her face, and blotting out the light?
>
> You wish to know the reason? Well, not very far away,
> There's the sound of little voices – 'tis the children at their play.
> Just peep inside! There's Daddy with the baby on his knee,
> And there's Mother in the corner looking on contentedly.
>
> Many times she's seen the picture; many times her eyes o'erflow,
> And she longs with deepest longing that such joy she, too, might know;
> Yet the years pass on unheeding, only God knows what she feels,
> Gives her needed grace and courage as before His throne she kneels.
>
> That is why you see her smiling as she passes on her way,
> Taking up her cross and gladly following Jesus day by day.
> There are many lonely women whom no earthly lover kissed.
> But God loves them, loves them dearly, for they're just His treasures missed.

As I improved and became more aware of my disabilities, I was determined to learn to walk again. But resources at the Physiotherapy department were stretched. After they had put me through some basic exercises they said I was not responding well enough. They had other, younger patients to help. So we hired the services of Barbara Taylor, a private physiotherapist. I wanted to walk, I told her, so that I would not be such a burden on others. I set myself the goal of walking to the toilet.

'Then that's what we'll aim for,' she told me.

What she did not tell me was that she had little more hope than the hospital physiotherapists that I would walk again. But she gave me no inkling of it at the time. She came twice a week and we worked and worked. What a professional she was! She shouted and she encouraged; she pushed me that little bit further when I thought I could do no more; but she made sure at every step that there was never in any real danger to my health.

Barbara was amazed at my progress. I could never do it absolutely unaided, but with someone by my side to steady me, and with the help of a tripod, I walked to the toilet for the first time since my stroke. I had achieved my goal. It was a year to the day since I had started my sessions with her.

Over the next years Douglas and I struggled on together, and along with the frustrations and disasters there continued to be triumphs. Among the minor disasters was the time a helpful canvasser cheerfully pulled

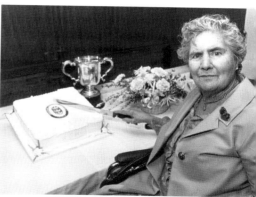

Celebrating 21 years of the WGH League, 1988

me out of the car she had transported me in to vote, not realising how restricted my mobility was. I came crashing to the ground and landed on my arm. When David arrived that evening he didn't like the look of the swelling above my wrist and took me into Casualty. An X-ray revealed a fracture and I spent the next six weeks in plaster, which limited my mobility still further. However, the candidate I voted for did get elected, so at least the vote was not wasted.

Another, more serious, disaster was in 1983, coming home from a celebration dinner to mark the centenary of the granting of the Hull Royal Hospital's charter at the Guildhall. A car swerved across our path as we approached Anlaby Square. Douglas just managed to avoid it, but we crashed into a bollard. Fortunately both of us were wearing seatbelts, but the car was a write-off, I broke my sternum and, most unfairly, Douglas had his licence taken away on account of his age, and because he had never taken a driving test. He was not to be allowed to drive again until he had taken lessons and passed the current-day test.

This was a most cruel thing: the accident was entirely the fault of the other driver; Douglas had been driving with an unblemished record for sixty years; and the ban dealt a severe blow to his independence. He persisted valiantly with a series of lessons, but his confidence had suffered and eventually he was forced to admit that he would never drive again. The days when he would help me into the car and we could just get to wherever we wanted to go under our own steam were over. It was a terrible, terrible shame. In time my sternum healed, but I think he never fully recovered from this blow to his self-esteem.

But with effort, taxis and the help of friends we did manage to get out for meals, attend special functions of the societies I belonged to and even go on holidays with the Disabled Christian Fellowship. With David's help I managed on two or three occasions to climb the stairs of the house and relish the unfamiliar sensation of seeing the upstairs bedroom, study and bathroom once again; however, since the stairs were steep and slippery I had to resort to a rather more undignified descent – sitting on the steps and easing down on my bottom, one tread at a time. But it was a triumph of its kind.

Another triumph, a great one, was my return visit to Malta at the request of the George Cross Island Association – which was only made possible with the heroic help of Marianne Tansey who accompanied us. Douglas came too and was able to see all the sights I had so often described to him. And I met again, among many others, Lieutenant Freddy Plenty, whom Eric Doyle had caught me spoonfeeding forty years before.

Eric Doyle had written short letters of encouragement and support since my stroke. He suffered from severe arthritis which kept him from doing the things he wanted to do now he was retired from the university. It was not long before I had news through a mutual friend, Peggy Evans, that Eric had moved into a nursing home. After that, his letters became far less frequent.

At the end of 1983 I had sad news of the other Eric in my life, through the Reverend Norman Hutchinson, whom I had first got to know when I was at the Kent and Sussex. He wrote to tell me that Eric Wells had died. Eric was seventy-five, almost exactly my own age. I felt I should write to John Wells, who was by now a well-known satirist and writer, famous at the time for his *Private Eye* column 'Dear Bill'. John was my godson, and I had kept my silence so long. I sent a letter early the next year, explaining who I was and regretting that 'due to circumstances beyond my control' I had been unable to fulfil the duties of a godmother.

He wrote back almost immediately:

Dear Mina
Thank you very much for your letter which arrived here this morning via the BBC and my agents. It couldn't have come at a better time. Yesterday was the day we buried my father's ashes. I was feeling very lost and a link like that with the past is a wonderful comfort.

I don't know how long it is since you were in touch with the family – I remember both of them talking about you with affection – but Mum died nearly 25 years ago, very suddenly, of a heart attack, very cheerful to the last minute. I told her in the ambulance on the way to the hospital she wasn't to go converting the doctors and she smiled and said if she did it wouldn't be her that did it but the Lord.

Pop had a wonderful life, marrying again very happily in 1962, much loved by his congregation at Tunbridge Wells (after Teddington) then at Eastbourne and finally as Rural Dean of Bognor. He'd been a bit gloomy over the last eighteen months because of minor strokes that robbed him of a lot of his natural confidence but the last time I saw him in hospital he was altogether his old self and to die in his sleep at home was all he would have asked.

I'll ring David when I can but would also love to see you and I hope we can arrange it soon. Are you ever in London?
Love, John

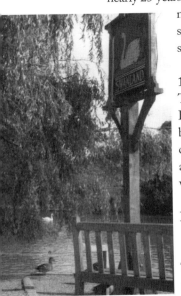

The pond at Swanland

The following October he wrote to tell us that he would be coming north and wondered if he could visit us – 'I'd love to see you both…if you could face having me'. We were overjoyed at the idea and he spent a week with us before setting off on a walking holiday around North Yorkshire. He reminded me so much of his father. They both spoke fluent French and they loved to go off walking together. It was so good to talk to him. I was able to tell him the full story of my friendship with his parents, and he was able to tell me much of what had happened in the intervening years.

A card arrived from him postmarked Flamborough a few days later, saying how good it was to talk about the old days. Three days on, another arrived from Pickering, thanking us for our hospitality and kindness. We exchanged news every Christmas for the next few years. He would let us know what work he was up to, and always expressed his concern for us and his interest in David's career.

David had been playing Aslan in *The Lion, the Witch and the Wardrobe*, both on tour and at the Westminister Theatre in London. When it arrived at the Palace Theatre in Manchester we even got to see the production – with the help of Marianne and Christopher Tansey and one of the Gibbs' sons, Malcolm. That November, 1987, we sent out our Christmas newsletter, which described our continuing struggle to keep our independence and the various difficulties which we had, with the Lord's help, managed to overcome. A few weeks later we were delighted to receive a card and letter from John. He wrote:

> My dear Douglas & Mina
> Thank you both for your Christmas letter and despite your bad news your faith and courage is a great inspiration.
>   I may be working with Ronald Mann at the Westminster Theatre later in the year: as I was walking through the foyer I saw a picture of your David and Ron talked about him with great admiration for the understanding he had brought to his work in the C S Lewis play.
>   God bless you both
>   Love, John
>
> PS I've just finished doing an adaptation of *Alice in Wonderland* at the Lyric Hammersmith and am trying to write a story about the Wesleys.

Douglas was suffering dreadfully from a varicose ulcer which had opened up on his ankle. This was part of the 'bad news' John referred to in his letter. It became agony for him to put any weight on his foot. He was tireless in his devotion to me, but he was in his mid-eighties now and not able to look after me entirely on his own.

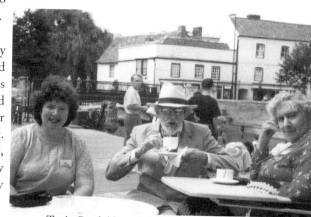

Tea in Cambridge on holiday with Pat and Douglas, 1989

We were already having some private nursing help. David persuaded his father to arrange some more. It was expensive and, after our years of independence together, unavoidably intrusive, but among the new carers was one who struck up an immediate rapport with us, and was responsive to our every need. Her name was Pat Glaholm. It was not only myself but Douglas too who now required a degree of care. Pat turned out to be a real treasure: just the right kind of person arriving in our lives at just the right time. She was to be an immense source of comfort and support for many years to come. Another answer to prayer.

Pat was the friend with whom, in 1989, on a Disabled Christian Fellowship holiday, I returned to the Round Church in Cambridge – to show her and Douglas the place where Douglas Johnson caused me such heartbreak all those years before.

Not long after I had come out of the coma caused by my stroke, I remember having a kind of vision.

I was looking up through the hospital window. It seemed to me that the sky was full of neon lights. I looked at them and saw that they were letters of the alphabet. Then, as I watched, they grouped together, and I read:

I AM THE LORD YOUR HEALER.

I said, 'Thank you, Lord. Oh, I do thank you. I claim that promise. You are my healer.'

To this day I believe it. I believe that the Lord is healing me.

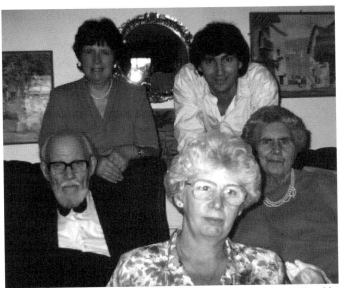

Celebrating our Ruby Wedding with Pat Glaholm, Marianne Tansey and David, 1990

17

...But Triumphantly

And death shall have no dominion
Romans 6.9

> It is with much sadness that I have to tell you Douglas passed away on
> Saturday 17 April at three o'clock in the morning. The funeral was held at
> Trafalgar Street Church today.
>
> But we do not grieve for we know we have the sure hope of meeting him
> again and rejoice that he is now free from pain and stress. Absent from the
> body, present with the Lord. He has now received the welcome, *My good and
> faithful servant, enter now into the joy of your Lord. Receive the crown of life for
> ever more.*

This was the letter David helped me compose after the death of my beloved
Douglas in 1993. We sent it out to all who knew Douglas but who were unable
to get to the funeral which took place on the twenty-second of April.

Around a hundred people were present at Trafalgar Street for the service that
Thursday. Our friend Peter Nelson, an member of the church, had agreed to
conduct the service. First, he led the congregation in this prayer: 'We have come
to honour the memory of a dear man, to support one another at a time of loss,
and to seek help for the future, especially for Mina and David. We come from
different backgrounds, different walks of life, but we pray that you will help each
one of us to fulfil our purpose for being here today. Amen.'

We sung the hymn I had chosen to begin the service, *Morning has Broken*.
Then, guided by a few notes, but speaking from the heart, Peter delivered his
tribute to Douglas:

> We've come today to honour the memory of Douglas. Douglas was born just
> after the turn of the century. When he was sixteen he lost both his parents
> within a few weeks in an epidemic of influenza. So he moved from the South
> of England up to Lincolnshire to stay with relatives there, and then went to
> Hull where he eventually got a job with an estate agent. He spent most of the
> rest of his life here.
>
> When he was in his twenties something happened that had a profound
> effect upon him. Like many at that time he attended church. But he found the

services unhelpful and uninspiring. Then somebody gave him a New Testament, and Douglas read it as he travelled to and from work on the bus each day. Reading all the way through the Gospels he came to accept the Christian faith in a way he had not done before. He accepted the teaching of Jesus as his code for living. He believed that Jesus not only died but rose again and ascended into heaven. He committed his life to Jesus and sought His forgiveness and His help from that day onwards. There was no preacher; there was no pressure. He just quietly read the life and record of Jesus.

Having found this new faith, he then found the company of others of like faith. They met together regularly and eventually purchased this very church, here at Trafalgar Street. It used to belong to the Baptists, but it was purchased by that independent fellowship of those believing in Jesus through the Bible.

That was in the late Thirties. Soon after the purchase of this church, war came and Douglas joined the Royal Marines. He joined as a conscientious objector, which meant that he wasn't involved in combat, but it didn't mean that he wasn't subjected to danger. He served on the European field and we are grateful that he returned to us alive.

He came back to Hull, to his work as an estate agent, to his flat at Eldon Grove, and to the fellowship of this church, when the second great event in his life took place. He met Mina Staerck – who had come to Hull to train in the teaching of nursing – and he fell in love with her, and she with him. They married, and to their great delight David was born to them.

Mina shared the same personal Christian faith that Douglas did, and their life together was centred on the Lord in prayer, and in serving Him together. A favourite verse was from Acts chapter seventeen: 'In Him we live and move and have our being.' In Him, we. In Him, we two. Douglas and Mina. Together.

They purchased a house in Eldon Grove, and used it as somewhere people could come and visit, or stay and receive Christian hospitality and help; and over the years a great many people, I know, found Christian succour through the open door and the warm invitation to Eldon Grove. I well remember, shortly after I came to Hull, enjoying their Christian hospitality, their kindness and generosity. During all this time, Douglas was supporting Mina in her teaching of nurses, as well as diligently carrying out his own work.

After retirement they moved out to Swanland. Then, as we know, Mina became ill. She suffered a stroke. This has been an enormous trial for her and for Douglas and for all those who are close to her. But love has triumphed in it. Douglas's love for Mina has triumphed in the way he cared for her; Mina's love for Douglas has triumphed in her continual concern for him, and her appreciation of him; and David's love for them both, and theirs for him; love that we have all shared – those of us who

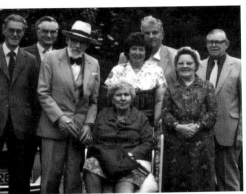

Douglas's 90th birthday with Peter Kemp, Peter Nelson, Pat and John Glaholm, Grace and Ken Gibbs

have kept in touch and visited. Love given and received: that love has triumphed. What has been in many ways a very difficult time has also been a time in which many of us have been brought closer together – not least Douglas and Mina themselves – and both of them to Jesus their Saviour. On numerous occasions, Douglas would tell me how truly precious were the times that he and Mina spent reading the scripture and praying together.

I cannot adequately describe Douglas's fine qualities. He endeared himself to everybody who met him. He was gentle, kind, courteous and thoughtful. These are very rare qualities. He was always scrupulously honest. He was always very appreciative: I'm sure you can hear him now, wanting to say to us, thank you – thank you to Mina for her love, to David for all his care, and to all those who have helped over the years.

He took a great delight in simple pleasures. He was also very interested in all new things, new inventions. And there was a twinkle about him – a real twinkle. He was full of life.

At the same time he managed his affairs well – even in these last years. He's been enterprising. He's been resourceful. I shall not forget Mina and I being rather concerned for him when, just a couple of years ago, he wanted to put up a new roof on the garden shed. But despite the fact he was approaching ninety, and was no longer so steady on his legs, he was determined to do it. And he did, and made an impressively thorough job of it. This was typical of his enterprise, his resourcefulness.

In looking after Mina he has won the admiration of us all – in his love, his devotion, his determination to keep going, and to keep loving.

Douglas's last letter to me

Douglas was also modest. He would not like to hear me speaking about him in this way. He would want to say that all these qualities derive not from himself, but the One to whom he committed himself nearly seventy years ago. He would say: my love for Mina, my love for you all, my integrity, my manner of life, cannot be disentwined from my devotion to my Lord in heaven. Indeed it was to Him that he looked for strength. Many times when I visited him it was this prayer he wanted: that he might be given strength from his Lord to keep going. And indeed it was into the hands of his Lord that he committed himself and Mina in hospital early last Saturday morning. Together we prayed for the Lord to look after him, to take him and to look after Mina.

So Douglas was a gentle man. More than that, he was a Christian gentleman. We shall miss him. We can draw inspiration from his life among us.

Peter Nelson paused for a moment of silence. Then announced the next hymn, *My Song is Love Unknown,* which had been one of the hymns at our wedding:

My song is love unknown, my Saviour's love to me
Love to the loveless shown that they might lovelier be.
O, who am I, that for my sake
My Lord should take frail flesh and die?

David had offered to give the reading. It was the one thing above all he felt he could contribute to his father's memory at the funeral. Now, as the rest of the congregation resumed their seats, he moved from his place by my side at the front of the church and went to stand at the podium. I had asked him to read Psalm 28:

Unto thee will I cry, O Lord my rock; be not silent to me: lest, if thou be silent to me, I become like them that go down into the pit… The Lord is my strength and my shield; my heart trusted in Him, and I am helped: therefore my heart greatly rejoiceth; and with my song will I praise Him. The Lord is their strength, and He is the saving strength of His anointed. Save thy people, and bless thine inheritance: feed them also, and lift them up for ever.

Kenneth Gibbs, who had been a friend of Douglas since the 1930's, stood to lead the congregation in prayer, and the service ended with another of my favourite hymns, *Great is Thy Faithfulness.*

Great is thy faithfulness! Great is thy faithfulness!
Morning by morning new mercies I see;
All I have needed thy hand hath provided.
Great is thy faithfulness, Lord, unto me.

The next few months were hard, trying to come to terms with the loss, finding the strength to keep going. Especially difficult were the times when I would forget that Douglas had really gone. I might turn to where his chair was beside me, wanting to share a sudden thought, and find the chair was empty, or at night call out to him to give me some assistance in the loving way he always did – but of course it would be Pat or Kathryn who came, and not my beloved Douglas. I would dream of him, and he always seemed so alive to me then, smiling down at me, talking to me. Whenever I woke, the realisation that he was no longer there took time to sink in once again.

But Pat and Kathryn, her daughter, and my other helpers were so good and understanding. Peter Nelson, and Ken and Grace, came at least once a week to see that I was adjusting to the new situation, and to give me precious Christian fellowship.

David kept a close watch on how things were going and made sure I had everything I needed. Before Douglas died I used to go into Castle Hill Hospital for respite care every couple of months. As soon as the hospital received news of his death, they informed me that they could no longer allow me to do this. I would have to make alternative arrangements. This made things difficult. David was trying to eke out my remaining funds for as long as possible, but I needed twenty-four-hour care, which was not cheap. And Pat and Kathy would have to have a break from time to time.

He looked around and made enquiries of several local nursing homes and towards the end of June we decided on trying one called Ferriby House. On my arrival, there was a letter waiting for me. It was from David to welcome me to my two-week stay.

Dear Mother

Today is 23 June. I have been conscious all day that it would have been Father's birthday if he were still alive. I'm sure it must have been on your mind. I hope it did not make you too sad. The little card you sent me a few weeks ago entitled 'Death is Nothing at All' is very comforting, especially where it says:

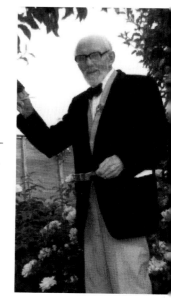

Laugh as we always laughed
at the little jokes we enjoyed together.
Let my name be ever the household word that it always was.
Let it be spoken without affect,
without the trace of a shadow on it...
Why should I be out of mind because I am out of sight?

Father has certainly not been out of my mind recently – and especially today. In a funny way, I have felt as though he has been looking after me in the weeks since he died.

You have been marvellous in dealing with so great a loss. But I know that you understand what the writer is getting at with the words:

I am waiting for you, for an interval,
somewhere very near, just around the corner.

I hope you can continue to take comfort from these words during your stay at Ferriby House and feel that Father is really not too far away. I hope too that the unfamiliar surroundings will soon become a place of enjoyment, and the unfamiliar faces will soon become friends.

It won't be long before you'll be back at home and enjoying all the things you can only really enjoy there.

I'll be writing to you again very soon.

All my love to you

David

In the September of that year, several of my friends came to the house to attend a small service we held for the scattering of Douglas's ashes in the garden. David could not be there as he was working abroad at the English Theatre in Frankfurt. But Pat was there with her husband John and Kathryn. Ken and Grace Gibbs were there with their son Malcolm, and so were other old friends of the family: Rupert Griffin, Doris Jackson, Dorothy Peers, Cherry Robinson. Peter Nelson again led the service. He began with a prayer.

'Oh, Lord, we seek your presence with us now, and your help in what we are about to do. It brings back to us our sadness, our sense of loss, but we pray that you will cheer us with your presence, and with the knowledge that Douglas is with you in heaven, and that one day we shall see him again and be together again. So, Lord, do please help us, because we pray, Lord Jesus, in your name. Amen.'

He turned to the Gospel of John and read aloud, 'For God so loved the world that He gave His only Son, that whoever believes in Him shall not perish but have eternal life. *Shall not perish but have eternal life,*' he repeated to allow those words to sink in. Then he led us in another prayer.

'Lord, we thank you for the earthly body of Douglas in which he lived his life among us. We know, Lord, that his body was made of the elements of the earth. Therefore we return it to the earth. Help us honour his memory respectfully and carefully. Cheer us with your presence. As we go outside, may we know that you are with us and close to us, and may we feel within ourselves that one day we shall see Douglas again, that we shall be with him again. Amen.'

We went into the garden where John had planted three rose bushes in memory of Douglas. We had chosen his favourite rose. It was peach-pink in colour and has a beautifully delicate scent. The name of the rose was Peace.

We poured the ashes around the base of the rose bushes. Together, we prayed the Lord's Prayer. And Peter concluded with the words of peace:

The peace of God which passes all understanding, keep our hearts and minds in the knowledge and love of God. May the blessing of God Almighty, Father, Son and Holy Spirit, be with us and remain with us always. Amen.

18

Day by Day

Do not be anxious about tomorrow,
for tomorrow will be anxious for itself
Matthew 6.34

Tuesday 14 September 1993

It is with Kathryn's help that I'm able to keep this diary. She sets up the cassette recorder in front of me when I think I've got something to say and starts it recording. Kathryn has been such a help, such a blessing. And her two little girls are so lovely. It's always a joy when they come to see me.

I've been out in the garden twice over this last week. I've spent the afternoon and had tea out there under the parasol. The apple trees are blossoming and the plum tree also has fruit, and we've had quite a few raspberries, so it seems that the garden is producing. The ballerina tree is full of fruit. By the time David returns to England, the apples will be ripe to eat.

The garden at the back overlooks fields, some of which have been put to use by a riding school set up in the old farm over there. Two days ago Kathryn's children and I set off to see the horses. We took bits of apple for them.

Yesterday I was at Swanland House. I go there twice a week – Mondays and Fridays – for day care, and a bath since I can no longer get upstairs to have a bath at home. It's just at the top of the road and near enough for Pat or Kathryn to take me round in the wheelchair.

The staff there were asking after David, so I was able to bring them up to date about his job in Frankfurt. Unfortunately, I was unable to have a bath yesterday because their electric machine for raising and lowering the bath seat had broken down, but they are hoping to have it repaired for Friday.

Tuesday 26 October 1993

I arrived home yesterday from my two-week stay in the Hesslewood Nursing Home. I had a bath every night. A long lingering bath. I could soak and feel the aches and pains just fade away. It was most comforting.

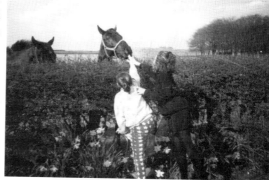

Lyndsey and Samantha feeding the horses

They were all very good to me. The food was excellent. Rather too good. I was inclined to eat more than I should, so I'm afraid I've put on some weight. But now I am home I'll do my best to keep to a strict diet to try and lose the surplus.

I felt a bit sad when I returned home. When I used to come back from my fortnight at Castle Hill, Douglas would be sitting there, and he would jump to his feet and take me into his arms and hug me and tell me how much he loved me, how much he had missed me. Now when I come in, the chair is empty, and it makes me sad. I long to see him.

Pat was behind me in the hall, and at the very moment I saw the empty chair, she said, 'Mina, there's a letter for you here from David.' So I sat down in my chair and I read it. It was such a comfort to me. He has so much of his father in him: his father's love and thought.

While in Hesslewood I thought of David often. I am so glad that Maureen is in Frankfurt with him now for a visit. They must make the most of these days and their love for each other. Such days are very precious. As I think back over my life with Douglas, I discover how precious those memories are. Above all, I know that his love will never fade. It is with me always.

Kathryn is with me this evening with her children, Samantha and Lindsey. They are so affectionate. They call me 'Nana Mina'. I count that a privilege. They are like grandchildren to me. They are beautiful, and do all sorts of wonderful things for me.

Behind the main building at Hesslewood there is a little menagerie of animals: two llamas, a white one and a brown one; a herd of deer; goats, rabbits, squirrels and the odd cat or two. When Kathryn and the children came to see me they were allowed to visit the menagerie and look at the animals. They were thrilled to do that.

In November they are having an open day at Hesslewood and there will be a bazaar, a sale of work of all the arts and crafts that are made there. During my fortnight there I attended the occupational therapy sessions. I found the musical movement helpful. We shrug our shoulders and make circles with our arms and lunge up and down and sideways.

Following that session we had a quiz, similar to the quizzes they have on TV. That first week, believe it or not, I won. We had it again the week after, and I won again. A voluntary helper runs these sessions. 'Well, you've done it again!' she said. I even got a little prize: a biscuit covered with chocolate called Boost. It was a happy time and it helped me to get to know some of the people. I enjoy that very much, having chats with them.

There was a gentleman there – of about sixty I should say – and we used to talk occasionally. One day as he was going out after tea I said, 'Good night, Peter.'

'Oh,' he said, 'you've remembered my name. That's very nice.'

And yesterday, when I was getting ready to go home, he came over and said, 'I believe you are going home soon?'

I said, 'Yes, I am.'

'Well, it's been nice knowing you,' he said. 'Will we see you again?'

'Yes, I think so,' I said. 'I'm coming back for the open day. What about you? When will you be going home?'

'Oh,' he said, 'I'm here for keeps.'

He lost his wife early last year. She was a diabetic and had gangrene of the legs and feet. He said how much he missed her. I said I could quite understand. 'I miss my husband too. But we have our memories.'

'That's right,' he agreed. 'That's what we must hold on to, isn't it?

Thursday 11 November 1993

I'm just drinking my nightcap. Horlicks. Kathryn is on duty. She makes a lovely drink. Not just Horlicks, but also a special milky coffee. She has a knack of giving it a tasty froth on the top.

I've started the Malta story for my memoirs. When it's completed Kathryn will send it off to David and he will type it into his computer and get it into shape.

Dictating today's date just now reminded me that it was Auntie Dagmar's birthday on 11 November, so my thoughts go back to those days when she always had a special dinner party. I remember on one occasion she made a table decoration – a cascade of poppies, spilling out over the table. This was to mark Armistice Day.

I wonder if they celebrate Armistice in Frankfurt, where David is working at the moment. It would be interesting to know.

The weather is changing. It is very cold.

I had an unexpected visitor yesterday. Stanley Wright. Douglas and I used to extend our hospitality to members of the Christian Police Association who were living in Hull. Stanley was one of their leaders. Then, after many years here, he moved to Scotland. He lives about forty miles north of Inverness. He had a lot to tell me. We talked about the time we first met, when I was at the School of Nursing and he arrived with his son who was twelve years old then and who is now in America. I got to know Stanley and his wife and his daughter very well.

Our talk brought back memories of so many things, so many people we had met. The CPA used to have gatherings in different people's houses, and they came to Eldon Grove several times. Stanley referred to those days. I was just sad that Douglas was not here to see him, because he liked Stanley very much. They will meet in glory.

Tuesday 16 November 1993

I have just finished the memoirs of Malta. Kathryn doesn't want to send the cassette to David through the post in case it gets lost. She will be keeping it here until he comes home and can take it with him. I filled both sides of the ninety-minute tape, so he should find it a useful account of what happened to me there during the war.

We have had some wintry weather in the past few days. Lots of rain. The wind has taken off the roof of the shed and damaged part of the utility room roof. Kathryn's husband, Richard, was able to fix them for the time being. He says they will need doing properly when David gets back and comes up here to visit.

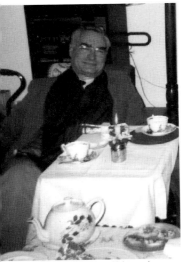

Peter Nelson enjoying a 'fairy tea'

It will be Peter Nelson's fifty-fifth birthday on Saturday, but since he cannot come on that day Kathryn and I are preparing a tea party for him on Thursday. With his heart condition, Peter is having to lose a little weight. He has to be careful what he eats, so we are preparing a 'fairy tea'.

A fairy tea is a special low-calorie tea. Three secrets are involved in making it. We have some wholemeal dough proving and shortly Kathryn will be baking it in the oven. When the bread has been turned out and allowed to cool, we shall slice it extremely thinly. That's the first secret of a fairy tea. The second secret is to spread a little butter on the bread, and then scrape most of it off again. Then instead of a filling – this is the final secret – you just use your imagination. You see, in your imagination they can be filled with whatever you wish – with no danger of adding any calories at all!

Friday is Hesslewood's open day. God willing, and the weather being favourable, Kathryn will take us there. All the arts and crafts will be on show. I shall have to take some money with me in case there are things I want to buy.

Saturday 20 November 1993

David will be preparing to come home to London from Frankfurt. He has been there for the last three months. He will be returning to Maureen. They'll be glad to be together again. What a lot they will have to tell each other.

Maureen will be able to bring him up to date on my news, because I was able, last Tuesday, for the first time in ages, to have a conversation on the phone. Kathryn had succeeded in finding a way to connect my hearing-aid box with the telephone. I had quite a chat with Maureen and she was going to phone David that evening and tell him all about it.

On Thursday we held the birthday party for Peter Nelson. He came at half-past five and what a happy time we all had. Kathryn had prepared a marvellous tea. He was delighted. Kathryn's two girls were here, and at the end they sang,

> Thank you for the world so sweet
> Thank you for the food we eat
> Thank you for the birds that sing
> Thank you Lord for everything

The next day I was at Swanland House for the day. Nothing special happened. I read a book, that was the main thing. But I had a long chat with one of the patients whom I have got to know. She had been away in hospital in Anlaby to have a hip replacement. Her name is Nan Holland. Years ago she was a nurse in Newcastle. That was one of the hospitals I used to go to when I examined the nurses.

I'm thinking about what I'm going to say in our Christmas newsletter. David will help me with that. There will be fewer people to send to. More of our friends have died in the last twelve months. The letter about Douglas's death which we mailed out in April to everyone on the list has been returned from several places as 'not known at this address'.

Saturday 1 January 1994

I am staying in Hesslewood again for the Christmas period.

David and Maureen came up from London on the twenty-eighth and have been in to see me every day. David brings the tape recorder in so that I can record more material for the memoirs. Now that most of the story has been told, he is getting me to fill in some of the gaps.

My room has a view of the field and wooded hedgerow bordering the place where the nurses and visitors park their cars. Yesterday we saw a deer and his doe edging out of the trees and towards the parked cars. Maureen was delighted. She is lovely.

Today they walked from Swanland to see me because the licence on the Metro expired at the end of December and we have decided not to renew it. It took them fifty minutes, and they said they enjoyed it, though it seems a long way to me.

The car is in the garage most of the time now, and David thinks it may be best to try selling it. My care is expensive – especially places like Hesslewood – and he is looking for ways to save money where he can. Jane, the senior nurse here, said she might be interested in buying it if she could raise the cash. Her car is becoming more and more unreliable.

During the years I have needed care – this is the fourteenth year since my stroke – I have met again many of the nurses whom I trained at Western General and then at the Hull School of Nursing. Jane is one of them. I must say, they are all extremely good at their job!

Today, just as I was describing to David and Maureen – for the memoirs – the time I wanted to take up the sister tutor diploma course and the matron did not want to let me go, another of the nurses I trained popped in to see me. Her name is Carol. I discovered only yesterday, New Year's Eve, that she works here at Hesslewood.

I remembered her clearly. When I ran the preliminary training school at Western General and later at the Hull School of Nursing, I believed in taking the trainee nurses on the wards and letting them learn by

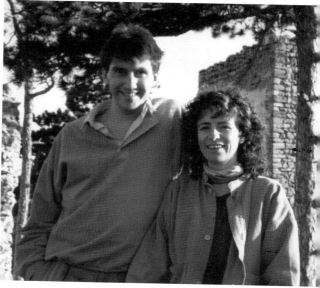

David and Maureen

helping out there, watching the nurses at work and even lending a hand where they could – bathing patients, perhaps, and making beds.

Carol was one of a batch of trainees I had arranged should go over to the hospital. I would send them across to the head sister of a department who would allocate them to the wards. I would go round a few hours later to see how they were getting on.

This particular girl, Carol, was extremely young looking. She was tiny and looked about twelve years old. I arrived at the chronic male ward she had been allocated to, in the old part of the hospital, and asked the male charge nurse, 'Where's the little nurse I sent?'

'In the bathroom,' he said.

I went along to the bathroom, and there she was. There was an old man in the bath, and she was crying. She appeared frightened. 'What's the matter?' I asked her.

'I don't know what to do,' she wailed. 'I've never seen a man before – like this.' And she indicated the poor old man, naked in the bath. She was scared – and he was shivering with embarrassment and cold.

'Go back to the ward,' I told her. 'Put your cloak on and go back to the school. I'll see to this. But you go back straightaway. It's all right. You're not staying here. I'm going to have a word with the nurse.'

So off she went, and I went to see the charge nurse.

'What do you mean by leaving that young trainee with an old man?' I asked him. 'I don't suppose she's ever seen a naked man before. These girls are too young to be left on their own.'

'They've got to learn, haven't they?' he replied. 'Isn't that why you send them over here?'

'Yes,' I said. 'But they won't learn this way. They come to assist, to learn by observing. You should have been in there with her, demonstrating the proper way to deal with an elderly male patient. You've probably put her off nursing for good. Well, you'll have to get on with him yourself now. And in future you won't be getting any more of my nurses.'

So saying, I left the ward and went back to the school to see how the little nurse was. She was so relieved and grateful to me, though really the situation should never have arisen. I've never forgotten that incident, and she tells me now that she's never forgotten it either. It was such a shock to her. She thought she would never be able to succeed as a nurse. But she got through her exams with flying colours, and I wrote her a special letter of commendation because I felt she had done extremely well.

Though she looked so young, she must have been about seventeen at the time. She was ever such a pretty girl. She's ever so pretty now. But she's a woman now, of course.

As I said, I didn't know she worked here until last night. She's been on night duty. She does the ten o'clock rounds with the medicine, so she's seen me but usually I'm very sleepy by that time. But last night I noticed she was looking at me, and she said, 'You know, I was in your school.'

'Were you?' I said. 'Were you with Jane?'

'No. It was about twenty years ago. I was in your school the year you retired.'

'That was 1973.'

'Yes, that's right. I was there then. You trained me.'

Then she reminded me of the incident I've just described. Oh dear.

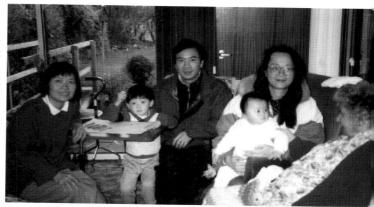

China has come to me: Viva visiting with her friends, 1995

It got me thinking a lot last night, remembering all the different nurses I trained.

Tuesday 8 February 1994

Last night I dreamed that David took me to his farmhouse in France. It was beautiful: except that I looked up at the wrought-iron staircase and wondered how I was going to get up there. I must have got up somehow because I remember being in the bedroom and lying down, thankfully, on a comfortable bed.

The night before, I was dreaming about Douglas. I dreamed he stood at the side of my bed. He said to me, 'I'd like to come into bed, dear.'

'Come in then, darling,' I said.

And he came in, and took me in his arms, and I cuddled him.

Oh, it was so real. It was such a disappointment when I woke up and found it was just a dream.

Sunday 1 May 1994

Now, on the Friday and Saturday of every week, I attend the Manor House residential home for day care. It's just five minutes away, down Woodgates Lane in our neighbouring village of Ferriby. I still go to Swanland House on Mondays, but Manor House is funded by the social services and therefore free of charge. Swanland House costs £15 a day. We pay £2.50 for lunch and tea at Manor House, and £6 to Dave Green, our excellent new taxi-driver, to take me there and bring me back.

My first day at Manor House happened to be 1 April, which we speak of as being April Fool's Day, but it was to turn out to be anything but that. I had an extremely rewarding day.

As I passed from the bathroom to the hall which leads to the dining room, I noticed a gentleman sitting in a chair near the door. Somehow there was something familiar about him. The next time I had to visit the bathroom, I took a good look at him as the nurse wheeled me past. Oh yes, I thought, I know him. I was sure it was Doctor Bradley, my old tutor from Hull University: the one who had played the violin for us at our engagement party in the summer of 1950.

'What is the name of that gentleman by the door?' I asked the nurse when we got into the dining room. 'Is it John?'

'No,' she said. 'I think it's Arthur.'

'It can't be.'

'Well, it's either Arthur or Sidney,' she replied.

'No,' I said. 'It must be John.'

'Do you know him?'

'I believe I do.'

'I'll go and find out. Where do you think you met him?'

'At the university – forty-five years ago. Just before I was married. He was my chemistry and physics tutor. '

'I'll ask him. Would he know your married name?'

'He might. He came to my engagement party.'

'Well, just in case, what was your maiden name?'

'Staerck.'

A few minutes later she was back.

'Yes,' she said. 'He does know you. And his name is John. Dr John Bradley.'

'That's right! I knew that was him!'

'Well, he remembers you, Mina. Would you like me to take you out there to chat with him?'

'Couldn't he come in here where it's warmer?'

'Yes, of course. He comes here once a week for his lunch, and that'll be along in ten minutes' time. We can sit you together. Would you like that?'

She pulled out a chair so that it was facing me and then went out and brought Dr Bradley in. Oh, wasn't he pleased! And so was I. We shook hands and he said, 'Oh, this is wonderful.'

'Yes, it is, isn't it?' I said, and we began reminiscing. We talked for an hour-and-a-half, all through lunch and afterwards. He told me about the other tutors who had been at the university when I was there. We went over what had happened to the other members of my group, how they had got on since, how their careers had progressed. We happened to have been served spaghetti that day. You can imagine us, chatting away and trying to grapple with the spaghetti at the same time. Each week now I shall be able to meet him and chat again. He lives in Ferriby and a neighbour transports him to Manor House, just for lunch.

The following week we met again.

He said to me, 'I've been looking forward to this.'

'So have I,' I replied, and we settled down for another good chat. He told me he had recently written a book about chemistry. In fact, our mutual friend Peter Nelson had helped him edit it and get it published. John and Peter had worked in the same department at the university before John's retirement. His book is called *Before and After Cannizzaro*. It seems that Cannizzaro was an important figure in the development of chemistry. Dr Bradley told me a bit about him.

'Cannizzaro was an Italian chemist,' he said, 'a Professor at Palermo and then at Rome. He was born in 1826 and, do you know, he lived on into the beginning of this century. It's strange to me to think that he was still alive when I was born – this great chemist who so revolutionised the science. He developed a method of synthesising alcohols which is called Cannizzaro's reaction and he discovered a white crystalline substance known as cyanamide. He demonstrated how to distinguish between atomic weight and molecular weight. Oh, he achieved so much, and he only died in 1910. Just think! I was two years old at the time.'

When Dr Bradley had been my tutor I had never really thought about his age. I just assumed he was older than me. And I think he had made the same assumption. 'You were born in 1908?' I queried.

'Yes, that's right.'

'So was I!' I exclaimed.

We both laughed at that.

The next Saturday we met again. This time, just as lunch was about to be served, a senior member of staff took us into a little room off the dining room.

'Now you can sit together here,' he said, 'and talk to your hearts' content.'

So we were able to have lunch together, away from the clatter and the chatter.

'Last week, you said you were born in 1908,' I said. 'But you didn't mention which month. I was born in March.'

'My birthday's in August,' he replied.

Again we went over old times. I asked him if he still played the fiddle. Did he remember my engagement to Douglas when he played so beautifully for us?

'Of course I remember,' he said. 'I can't play so easily nowadays. But, yes, I still pick it up and have a go from time to time.'

He told me about his family. He had two sisters, both of whom had died, and a little dog – a Yorkshire terrier called Ben – who had died too. I told him that all my brothers and sisters were dead: the last to go had been Jean in Canada the previous year. I was the only surviving member of that generation of my family, I told him, though I was still close to my niece Margaret Samuels, the one who had sent that note to Douglas before our wedding: 'I hear you are hoping to marry my aunt. You better look after her. If not you'll have me to deal with!'

Margaret still comes up from Seaford to see me, and writes to me regularly. She lives in the bungalow her mother, my sister Mary, and her father, Frank Goldsmith, lived in before they died.

On the card with the flowers for Douglas's funeral, Margaret had written, 'To Douglas in loving memory. You certainly kept your promise!'

John Bradley had a clear memory of Douglas from the engagement party. I told him that Douglas had died exactly a year ago – in fact, almost to the day. Tomorrow was to be the seventeenth of April. He told me how sorry he was.

So ended another session. Despite the fact that our conversation had ended sadly with remembering our lost ones, I'm so thankful to have the company of someone with whom to talk over those memorable times. And so, I think, is John Bradley. April Fool's Day this year was anything but that for us.

* * *

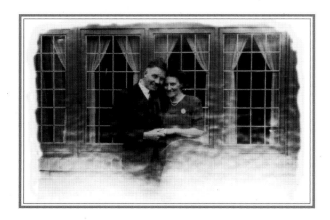

How wonderfully the Lord works. His ways are past finding out. But He knows best and He knows the end from the beginning.

I feel still that He has a certain work for me to do, and I am waiting for Him to reveal that work. I am old now and I am disabled. But He can use the disablement for His glory. I am willing and waiting to be used. I am waiting until that day when I shall meet the Saviour and know the reason why things happened as they did.

Looking back, I know why I was led to Yorkshire, to the University of Hull. I met a man whose name was Douglas Banks. We fell in love. And oh, what a wonderful man he was. He is now in glory. But I do not fret because I know I will see him one day – that glorious morning when we shall meet again and together we shall see the face of the Lord. In Him we live and move and have our being. We can trust in Him, knowing He will never fail us.

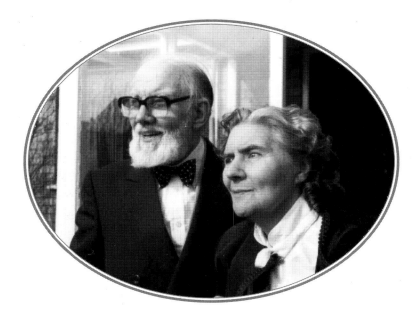